INDUSTRIAL HYGIENE SCIENCE SERIES

ERGONOMIC INTERVENTIONS TO PREVENT MUSCULOSKELETAL INJURIES IN INDUSTRY

American Conference of Governmental Industrial Hygienists

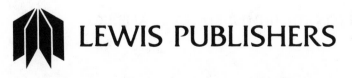

Library of Congress Cataloging-in-Publication Data

Ergonomic interventions to prevent musculoskeletal
  injuries.

  (Industrial hygiene science series ; no. 2)
  Papers presented at a symposium held Oct. 9–10,
1986.
  Includes bibliographies and index.
  1. Musculoskeletal system — Wounds and injuries —
Prevention — Congresses. 2. Human engineering —
Congresses. 3. Exercise therapy — Congresses.
4. Mechanotherapy — Congresses. 5. Disability
evaluation — Congresses. I. American Conference of
Governmental Industrial Hygienists. II. Series.
[DNLM: 1. Bone and Bones — injuries — congresses.
2. Human Engineering — congresses. 3. Muscles —
injuries — congresses. 4. Occupational
Diseases — prevention & control — congresses.
WE 500 E67 1986]
RD732.E74   1987   617.1   87-3177
ISBN 0-87371-103-3

LEWIS PUBLISHERS, INC.
121 South Main Street, P.O. Drawer 519, Chelsea, Michigan 48118

PRINTED IN THE UNITED STATES OF AMERICA

PREFACE

This volume contains most of the papers presented at a topical symposium entitled Ergonomic Interventions to Prevent Musculoskeletal Injuries in Industry. The chapters herein represent a cross-section of the papers presented.

The goal of the symposium was to bring together both researchers in the field of ergonomics and clinical and engineering practitioners for the purpose of 1) reviewing ergonomic methods for evaluating physically stressful jobs, 2) identifying conditions and personnel that increase the risk of occupational musculoskeletal problems, and 3) discussing contemporary approaches to controlling occupationally induced musculoskeletal disorders. Topics ranged from the discussion of the biomechanical cause of low back pain and carpal tunnel syndrome to how one organizes groups of people to identify, evaluate, and control such problems.

Several general themes were presented: 1) occupational musculoskeletal disorders are highly underreported in traditional OSHA logs, and state workers compensation data and new surveillance systems are needed, 2) knowledge of fundamental biomechanical principles is very helpful if one is to understand and prevent musculoskeletal disorders, and 3) several different organizational functions or disciplines in a large firm must be brought together to solve complex ergonomic problems — that is, a team approach appears to be best.

The attendees at the symposium rated the speakers and their topics very highly. This volume should serve as an excellent reference for those interested in this rapidly growing body of knowledge.

Don B. Chaffin, Ph.D.
Professor and Director
Center for Ergonomics
The University of Michigan

CONTENTS

ERGONOMIC
INTERVENTIONS
TO PREVENT
MUSCULOSKELETAL
INJURIES IN
INDUSTRY

CHAPTER 1

Quantifying Patient Capabilities to Return to Work

RICHARD E. JOHNS, Jr., M.D., MSPH

Rocky Mountain Center of Environmental Health, University of Utah, Salt Lake City, Utah

INTRODUCTION

Most workers who are injured on the job return to work after a reasonable healing period. For those who do not, the physician and rehabilitation team are faced with complex clinical, psychological, and legal dilemmas. Figure 1 demonstrates the multiple medical decisions required in removing or returning an injured worker to light, regular, or alternate duty, as well as the potential rating of permanent partial impairment.

Any type of return to work decision involves an appropriate matching of job requirements to physical abilities or limitations (Table I). Job requirements are further defined in terms of environmental conditions such as temperature, lighting, slippery surfaces, elevation, vibration, etc. Physical demand requirements, such as lifting, pulling, pushing, carrying, etc., should be evaluated by a trained job analyst who can determine load weights, posture, task frequency and duration, workstation layout, and body anthropometry. Several subjective work rating systems, such as the Model Standards Project[1] and GULHEMP[2] (G-general physique, U-upper extremities, L-lower extremities, H-hearing, E-eyesight, M-mentality, P-personality) systems, attempt to describe some of these job requirements. A two-dimensional strength prediction model has also been developed by The University of Michigan, Center for Ergonomics

1

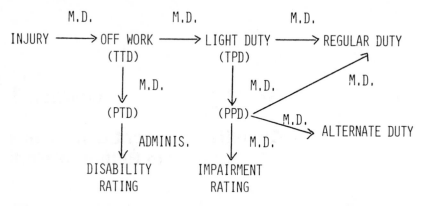

Figure 1.   Medical decision points in return-to-work or impairment cases.

to objectively rate the strength requirements and risks of various materials handling tasks. It is the objective evaluation of the job for which a physician has the least understanding to make informed decisions to return a worker to light or regular duty work.

Although a physician has the quantitative tools to evaluate joint or torso flexibility (e.g., bicycle ergometer or treadmill), eyesight (e.g., visual acuity tests), and hearing (e.g., audiometric evaluation), the quantitative determination of strength ability has been difficult to assess. A physician usually relies on the worker's subjective impression of whether he is capable of returning to a manual handling task without knowing himself what the actual job requirements and strength abilities are. A

TABLE I.   Matching Job Requirements with Physical Abilities or Limitations in Return-to-Work Decisions

Return-to-work Decisions

Job requirements

- Environmental conditions
- Physical demands

Physical abilities/limitations

- Strength
- Flexibility
- Aerobic capacity
- Eyesight
- Hearing

worker's strength should ideally be matched 1:1 to the actual force requirements involved for the job.

SIGNIFICANCE

The use of pre-employment strength testing methods has been promoted for the last decade as a means of controlling musculoskeletal injuries in the workplace. Chaffin and his colleagues have described in detail the methodology for conducting static strength tests in healthy individuals.[1-3] Keyserling[4] has described how to establish strength testing programs in industry. Although wide static strength variability exists among healthy individuals, Chaffin's data does provide some basis for determining "normal" human strength capability. Pre-employment strength testing as a worker selection technique should be considered after other engineering or administrative controls have been attempted as one method of preventing or reducing occupationally related musculoskeletal injuries.

The use of these same static strength testing methods to monitor the recovery of muscle strength among injured workers, however, has not been studied to our knowledge. The ability to quantify muscle strength recovery among injured workers in an industrial setting has great significance for workers, employers, physicians, rehabilitation specialists, and insurance carriers as further described below:

1. Workers who are injured on the job generally rely on a subjective sense of strength and pain improvement to assess their capability to safely return to a physically demanding job. As such, most workers will naturally tend to be conservative in the amount of healing time they feel is necessary for their specific injury. The ability to quantify strength recovery would help remove this subjective assessment in returning a patient to work or functional activity.

2. Employers generally do not want workers involved with manual materials handling to return to work until they have been released for regular duty by the treating physician. The quantification of strength recovery after injury could very well certify to an employer that the worker is fit for light or even regular duty sooner than the employee might subjectively determine that end point himself. Lost work time could thus be reduced and productivity preserved.

3. Physicians who treat industrial injuries could quantify their "clinical judgment" for strength improvement as they assess the patient's course of healing and eventual return to work. Such objective infor-

mation in a physician's hands would also help to sort out functional and emotional problems, potential malingerers, and reduce the potential for secondary financial gain among workers predisposed to such tactics.

4. Physical therapists or rehabilitation specialists would be able to provide an objective, quantitative profile of a patient's recovery during the course of treatment and therapy.

5. By reducing the time off for work-related injuries, it is hoped employers and their workers' compensation carriers would experience reduced compensation and medical care costs. Such savings would rightfully be passed on to employers in the form of reduced compensation insurance premiums.

The research required to establish such "strength recovery curves" for specific types of musculoskeletal injuries eventually could produce an invaluable tool to each of the above listed entities in managing both work- and nonwork-related injuries.

RESEARCH QUESTIONS

Our interest in the potential use of various pre-employment static strength testing models, as applied to an injured worker population, led us to conduct a short-term research study to answer the following questions:

1. Can strength recovery in an injured worker be quantified?

2. Does an injured worker regain static strength more rapidly than dynamic strength or vice-versa?

3. Does a work hardening/physical conditioning program accelerate strength recovery when compared to conventional therapy methods?

4. Does quantitative strength improvement correlate with pain intensity?

METHODS

Study Design

A case-comparison study was used with the patient serving as his own control.

Study Population

Twenty-five male patients were enrolled in the study between February and August 1986. Three females completed the program but were excluded from the data analysis due to small numbers. All patients had been referred to a local hospital-based work hardening program for chronic low back pain and were classified by worker compensation definitions as either temporarily totally disabled or temporarily partially disabled. All patients had been removed from pain medication prior to entering the program. Each individual was characterized by age and sex as well as the site, type, and date of injury. A pre-assessment evaluation included previous history and pertinent physical examination. Baseline flexibility, aerobic capacity, and pain intensity on a scale of 1–10 were completed on each patient. Each work hardening group consisted of 8–15 patients for a five-week therapy course. Patients were supervised by a trained physical therapist for four to six hours per day, five days per week. A progressive strength, flexibility, and aerobic fitness program was developed for each patient according to type of injury, physical ability, and symptom level. Back school and group therapy provided a positive environment to reinforce and maximize the patient's rehabilitation potential. All study subjects were required to discontinue use of pain medications, muscle relaxants, or other prescription drugs prior to entering the study. Only individuals who completed the entire five-week work hardening program were evaluated. Participation was strictly voluntary and individuals could choose to withdraw from the study without jeopardizing their benefit payments or continued participation in the work hardening program. Informed consent was obtained from each patient according to Institutional Review Board guidelines and Human Subject Committee approval at the University of Utah Health Sciences Center.

Strength Testing Procedures

Static and dynamic strength testing were evaluated in this study. Static strength was defined as muscle contraction with a body segment restrained against motion. Dynamic strength was defined as muscle contraction with movement of the body segment being tested. Static muscle strength was performed according to a modified procedure specified previously by Chaffin in the AIHA Ergonomic Guidelines for Static Strength Testing.[2] The guidelines call for a four- to six-second maximum voluntary exertion which we modified to prevent aggravation of pain or additional injury. The patient was required to generate only what he felt was a "safe" exertion against a fixed resistance without producing additional symptoms. Dynamic strength testing was performed according to psychophysical guidelines described by Snook[5] which allowed the patient to self-select increasing weights until he reached a "safe" maximum lift through at least a one-foot distance without additional symptoms.

The strength testing protocol for environmental conditions, examiner instructions, and strength testing positions is described in Appendix A.

As part of the pre-assessment evaluation, subjects were tested to establish baseline static and dynamic strength. They were then retested at the third and fifth weeks of the work hardening program. Pain intensity scores were obtained on the baseline and fifth week strength tests.

Equipment

Both static and dynamic tests were performed on the Statidyne strength testing system developed by Hoggan Health Industries, Draper, Utah. Muscle strength data in pounds were recorded by test position using an IBM compatible software program which prompted the examiner through the programmed set of strength tests. An IBM-PC with A-D interface capability was required to receive the load cell muscle force signal. The examiner recorded the peak and the three-second time-averaged exertions for static strength and the peak weight lifted for dynamic strength in each of the three test positions.

Results

Twenty-five male patients completed the entire five-week work hardening program and strength testing study. Two patients dropped out of the study due to pain or motivation problems. Group data for all 25 patients demonstrated beginning-to-end strength improvement for all six static and dynamic strength tests ($p < .01$, Wilcoxon Test). Strength regression analysis for the group data also demonstrated improvement for all strength tests ($p < .02$, Linear Regression) (Figures 2–4). The

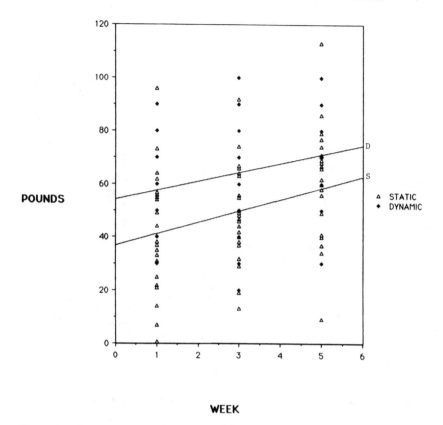

Figure 2. Static and dynamic strength regression analysis for arm lift (p < 0.02).

data is being analyzed currently to determine individual improvement based on linear regression analysis. A comparison group of pain-free "normal" individuals is being tested currently with the protocol to determine if learning effect contributed to strength improvement in the study population.

CONCLUSIONS

- It appears that progressive static and dynamic strength recovery can, in fact, be quantified and compared to normal worker strength for various test positions. The type of strength being tested, e.g., static, dynamic, isokinetic, etc., must be stated clearly and interpreted according to that specific type of test. Conclusions based on one type

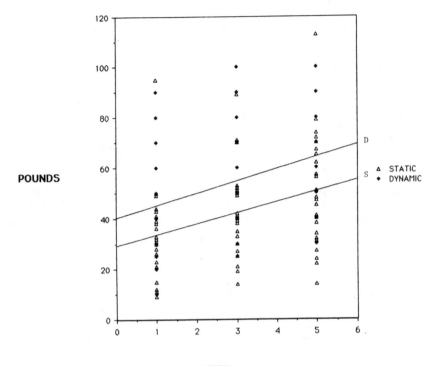

POUNDS

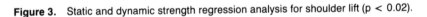

WEEK

Figure 3.   Static and dynamic strength regression analysis for shoulder lift (p < 0.02).

of strength test cannot be generalized to another type of strength test (e.g., static to isokinetic, etc.). The ability to quantify muscle strength in injured workers has the potential of establishing muscle "strength recovery curves" as increased numbers of patients are evaluated using these types of testing techniques.

- Both static and dynamic strength appear to have improved significantly with a work hardening intervention strategy. Both individual and group comparative data must be compared to a control group of non-injured workers to determine if learning effect has created a confounding bias.

- Normal data for various test positions must be obtained for comparing and quantifying return to work abilities. It would then be feasible for a clinician or rehabilitation specialist to strength test the patient and compare results to "normal" individuals for various test positions. The employee could also be matched appropriately to specific

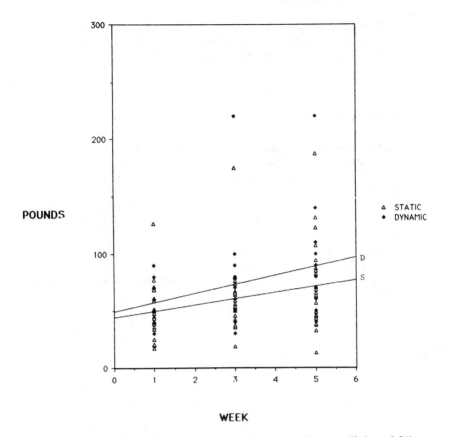

Figure 4. Static and dynamic strength regression analysis for torso lift (p < 0.01).

job strength demands to ensure safe lifting and to prevent aggravation of resolving symptoms or even reinjury.

- Further studies must be performed to determine if static or dynamic strength testing in injured workers is the most appropriate method of determining return-to-work strength abilities. Since the majority of manual materials handling activities involve dynamic lifting abilities, the testing of dynamic strength for return to work considerations requires further research.

- Since pain is a primary consideration in returning a patient to work and significantly affects a worker's ability to exert static or dynamic strength, further research efforts to correlate the effect of pain on strength is definitely warranted.

- We were unable to compare strength recovery between patients in a work hardening program and patients in a conventional physical therapy program. We are currently planning to extend this study to such a setting.

REFERENCES

1. Chaffin, D.B., G.D. Herrin and W.M. Keyserling: Pre-employment Strength Testing—An Updated Position. *J. Occup. Med. 20(6)*:403–408 (June 1978).
2. Chaffin, D.B.: Ergonomics Guide for the Assessment of Human Static Strength. *Am. Ind. Hyg. Assoc. J. 36*:505–510 (July 1975).
3. Stobbe, T.J.: The Development of a Practical Strength Testing Program for Industry. Unpublished Dissertation. Center for Ergonomics, University of Michigan (1982).
4. Keyserling, E.M. et al: Establishing an Industrial Strength Testing Program. *Am. Ind. Hyg. Assoc. J.* 41:730–736 (October 1980).
5. Snook, S.: The Design of Manual Handling Tasks. *Ergonomics 12(21)*:963–985 (1978).

CHAPTER 2

Postural Stress of the Trunk and Shoulders: Identification and Control of Occupational Risk Factors

W. MONROE KEYSERLING, Ph.D., LAURA PUNNETT, Sc.D. and
L.J. FINE, M.D.

Center for Ergonomics, University of Michigan, Ann Arbor, Michigan

INTRODUCTION

Awkward posture during work activities can be caused by the interaction of several factors, including poor workstation layout, inappropriate design or selection of tools and equipment, incorrect work methods, and/or the anthropometric characteristics of the worker. If not controlled, awkward postures can cause localized fatigue and contribute to the development of musculoskeletal disorders. Awkward postures are of particular concern for workers who perform repetitive jobs due to the frequency and cumulative effects of exposure.[1-3]

In a review of the effects of awkward posture, Van Wely[4] reported that trunk flexion (i.e., forward bending in the sagittal plane) was associated with reports of low back pain. Laboratory studies have demonstrated that non-neutral trunk postures such as flexion, lateral bending, and/or twisting increase the level of muscle fatigue and intra-discal pressures in the lumbar spine.[5,6] Epidemiologic studies have shown that lateral bending or twisting of the spinal column during manual materials handling activities (e.g., lifting, carrying, pushing, pulling) can increase the risk of low back pain.[2,7,8] Prolonged sitting has also been shown to be a postural risk factor associated with the development of back pain.[9]

Laboratory studies of nonneutral shoulder postures have shown that prolonged elevation of the arms (shoulder flexion or abduction) causes discomfort and local muscle fatigue.[5,10] A laboratory study by Hagberg[11] demonstrated that elevated arm work can cause acute tendinitis and pain at the shoulder. In studies of male industrial workers, use of the hands above shoulder height has been associated with increased chronic shoulder pain[12] and increased tendinitis of the shoulder rotator cuff.[13] Shoulder abduction and shoulder extension have also been cited as nonneutral postures related to the development of occupational thoracic outlet syndrome.[3,14]

The measurement and analysis of trunk and shoulder posture has two important occupational health applications: 1) evaluating a particular job to quantify postural stress and to identify specific causes (e.g., poor workstation layout) of awkward posture, and 2) obtaining exposure data for use in epidemiologic investigations of posture-related injury. Either application requires a complete and continuous description of the postures required to perform a job. Until recently, this has been a time-consuming and labor-intensive data collection activity, thus limiting the size and scope of epidemiologic studies. This problem has been overcome, however, through the development of a new system that utilizes videotape and a personal computer to document and reduce postural data.[15,16]

COMPUTER-AIDED POSTURAL ANALYSIS

The posture classification system in Figure 1 defines a menu of standard positions of the trunk and shoulders. This menu was developed by observing videotapes of work activities in several different manufacturing operations in order to establish a taxonomy of common work postures and by reviewing the literature to identify specific work postures associated with the development of fatigue and/or musculoskeletal disorders of the trunk and shoulders.[15] Conceptually, this classification system is similar to the Ovako Working Posture Analysis System (OWAS) developed by Karhu et al.[17] and the VIRA system developed by Kilbom et al.[18]

For a standing worker, the trunk is considered to be deviated from a neutral position if it is extended (bent backward), flexed (bent forward), bent sideways, or twisted more than 20 degrees from the vertical. Hyperflexion (i.e., forward bending of more than 45 degrees) is an addi-

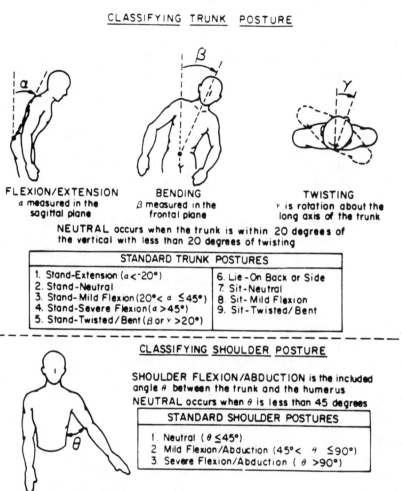

Figure 1. Standard postures of the trunk and shoulders.[15]

tional standard posture category. A similar rationale is used to classify the trunk posture of a seated worker.[15]

For either a standing or seated worker, the shoulder is classified as deviated from neutral if it is flexed or abducted more than 45 degrees. (This classification system does not consider the bearing of the upper arm or the humeral rotation angle.) Hyperflexion or abduction of the shoulder (i.e., raising the arm more than 90 degrees from the trunk so that the elbow is above shoulder height) is recognized as a standard posture category.[15]

The objectives of posture analysis are simple: 1) to determine the amount of time that a worker spends in each posture category, and 2) to determine the temporal aspects of posture changes. Operationally, however, postural analysis is difficult to perform for the following reasons:

1. Work posture can change very frequently, and a given posture may be held for only a fraction of a second. In order to analyze posture in real time, the observer must constantly focus attention on the worker and cannot be distracted to read a watch or to record posture and time data.

2. The analyst must simultaneously observe and record the position of three joints (the trunk, left shoulder, and right shoulder) which move independently. In real time, classifying and recording the postural status of multiple joints can quickly overload the observational and information processing capabilities of the analyst.

To overcome these problems, special procedures have been developed to assist the analyst.[15,16]

The first step in the posture analysis is to obtain a continuous video-tape recording of several work cycles for the job of interest. When making the tape, it is essential that the camera angle be chosen so that the joints of interest are not obstructed. In some situations, it is advisable to use more than one camera angle to record the job.

After returning to the laboratory, the next step is to reduce the data from the videotape. A procedure based on the industrial engineering time study methodology is used to collect postural data while viewing the videotape in simulated real time, i.e., the tape is played back at the same speed at which it was recorded. A personal computer (IBM-PC or compatible, equipped with a printer and two floppy disk drives) is used to assist the analyst in timekeeping and clerical tasks. The computer keyboard is used to enter data while the tape is played. To do this, each of the standard postures is assigned a key. Whenever the worker changes posture, the analyst strikes the key corresponding to the new posture. The value of the new posture and the time of the posture change (taken from the computer's internal clock at the time of the keystroke) are stored on diskette for subsequent analysis and archiving. Because the computer performs all clerical functions, the analyst can devote uninterrupted attention to the videotape. This is an essential feature due to the very short time (sometimes less than 0.25 seconds) between posture changes on a highly dynamic job.

To eliminate the need to observe multiple joints simultaneously, the tape is played one time for each joint of interest. Each analysis is performed on a common timescale, with zero corresponding to the start of the work cycle.

After data entry is completed, the computer generates a posture profile for each joint of interest. The profile provides basic descriptive statistics for postural activity (e.g., the total time spent in each standard posture during the work cycle, the minimum and maximum times spent in each standard posture, the number of times the posture was entered, etc.) An example of a posture profile for an automobile assembly job is presented in Table I.

POSTURAL RISK FACTORS—RESULTS OF A CASE-REFERENT STUDY

The system described above was used in a case-referent (case-control) study of automobile assembly workers to evaluate the relationships among postural stress and disorders affecting the trunk and shoulders. The goals of this study included developing a description of the postural requirements of jobs in the plant, and estimating the extent to which these postures contributed to the back and shoulder disorders that occurred in the plant. Cases included all workers who 1) reported to the plant medical department with a first trunk or shoulder injury and 2) met criteria for persistent pain on interview. Referents were workers selected randomly from the same departments of the plant who had not reported a trunk or shoulder injury and who did not report persistent pain on interview. Based on these criteria, 95 back cases, 79 shoulder cases, and 124 referents were identified and included in the investigation.[19]

One job was recorded on videotape and analyzed using the computer-aided system for each case (back or shoulder) and referent.

Descriptive statistics for time spent in nonneutral postures and the frequency of posture changes are presented in Table II for the trunk. Of the 219 workers, 185 (84%) had jobs that required mild flexion during some part of the work cycle, severe flexion was required of 112 workers (51%), and bending or twisting was required of 98 workers (45%). Several jobs required substantial static loads on the trunk muscles. Four jobs required workers to stand in mild trunk flexion for more than 45% of the work cycle, and one job required mild flexion for 80% of the cycle. Three jobs required severe trunk flexion for at least 45% of the cycle with one job requiring severe flexion for 74% of the cycle. Dynamic

TABLE I.   **A Computer-generated Posture Profile for the Trunk and Shoulders**[15]

JOB TITLE: Spotweld

TRUNK

POSTURE	FREQ.	MIN.	MAX.	MEAN	ST. DEV.	TOTAL
Neutral	3	1.3	39.1	14.4	21.4	43.2
Mild Flex.	1	11.1	11.1	11.1		11.1
Sev. Flex.	2	6.3	7.9	7.1	1.1	14.2
Twist/Bent	1	6.9	6.9	6.9		6.9

Posture Changes = 7
Cycle Length = 75.4

LEFT SHOULDER

POSTURE	FREQ.	MIN.	MAX.	MEAN	ST. DEV.	TOTAL
Neutral	5	4.0	27.5	11.3	9.3	56.5
Mild Flx/Abd.	4	1.0	6.8	4.7	2.7	18.8

Posture Changes = 9
Cycle Length = 75.3

RIGHT SHOULDER

POSTURE	FREQ.	MIN.	MAX.	MEAN	ST. DEV.	TOTAL
Neutral	4	2.6	39.5	14.6	16.8	58.4
Mild Flx/Abd.	3	4.4	7.5	5.7	1.6	17.1

Posture Changes = 7
Cycle Length = 75.5

TABLE II.   **Trunk Postures Required by the Jobs of 219 Automobile Assemblers, 95 Cases and 124 Referents**[19]

	N	Minimum	Mean	Median	Max.
Percentage of job cycle					
Trunk in mild flexion	185	0.2%	13%	9%	80%
Trunk in severe flexion	112	0.2%	11%	7%	74%
Trunk twisted or bent laterally	98	0.3%	6%	4%	35%
Frequency of posture changes/minute					
Change in any direction	219	0.7	7.2	6.7	18.5
Mild trunk flexions	185	0.2	2.4	2.3	7.2
Severe trunk flexions	112	0.3	1.4	1.1	5.3
Trunk twists	98	0.2	1.4	1.2	4.6

postural demands could also be high; one job required 18.5 changes in trunk posture per minute.[19]

The use of each nonneutral trunk posture was compared among cases and referents by computing cross-products odds ratios. Cases were approximately five times more likely than referents to work with the trunk in mild flexion for any length of time and almost six times more likely to work with the trunk in severe flexion or bent and twisted sideways. (See Figure 1 for reference standard postures.) Furthermore, the magnitude of the odds ratios increased with increasing length of exposure to each nonneutral posture. For both mild and severe trunk flexion, there was substantial increase in risk if the posture had to be maintained for more than 10% of the work cycle.[19]

Descriptive statistics for time spent in nonneutral shoulder postures and the frequency of posture changes are presented in Table III. All 203 workers had jobs requiring mild flexion or abduction of one or both shoulders. One hundred four workers (51%) were required to use severe flexion or abduction of at least one shoulder during the work cycle; the remaining 99 workers never used severe flexion or abduction. Several jobs involved substantial static loading of the shoulder muscles. Twelve workers were required to hold the left shoulder in mild flexion, and 12 workers were required to hold the right shoulder in mild flexion, for more than 50% of the work cycle. Dynamic demands were also high on some jobs, with as many as 34.7 changes in shoulder posture per minute.[19]

The use of nonneutral shoulder posture was compared among cases and referents by computing cross-products odds ratios and their approximate 95% confidence intervals. Cases were two to three times more likely than the referents to work with at least one shoulder in severe flexion. Cases a'so worked longer with each shoulder in severe flexion. Further-

TABLE III. Shoulder Postures Required by the Jobs of 203 Automobile Assemblers, 79 Cases and 124 Referents[19]

	N	Minimum	Mean	Median	Max.
Percentage of job cycle					
Left mild flexion or abduction	200	0.8%	24%	22%	82%
Right mild flexion or abd.	203	3.4%	28%	26%	81%
Left severe flexion or abd.	72	0.2%	8%	3%	66%
Right severe flexion or abd.	86	0.1%	8%	4%	43%
Frequency of posture changes/minute					
Left, either direction		0.9	10.0	9.5	26.7
Right, either direction		3.0	12.6	11.6	34.7

more, the magnitude of the odds ratios increased with increasing expo-sure time. These associations were stronger for the left shoulder than for the right.[19]

IMPLICATIONS ON WORKSTATION DESIGN

The results reported above suggest that non-neutral postures of the trunk and shoulders are a contributing factor to the development of injuries and disorders in these body regions. Jobs with significant pos-tural demands should be redesigned where feasible to eliminate postural stresses. General recommendations for workstation layouts that encour-age neutral trunk and shoulder postures are presented below.

Guidelines to Prevent Awkward Trunk Postures

In many work situations, awkward posture is caused by the excessive reach requirements of a specific task. For example, trunk flexion occurs when the reach target lies outside the arc illustrated in Figure 2a. The radius of this arc is the distance between the shoulder and fingers in a fully extended arm. Its center is the position of the shoulder when the trunk is in a neutral (i.e., fully vertical) posture. Task-related trunk flexion can usually be attributed to one of two causes: 1) reaching for an object that is lower than the height of the hands when standing with the arms fully relaxed (i.e., hanging vertically at the side of the body), or 2) reaching for an object that is too far in front of the body.

The above example illustrates the mechanical approach to workstation design. In this approach, the body is treated as a system of rigid links that are connected at joints. By adding up the sizes of each of the links, it is possible to determine where objects should be located so that they can be reached easily.[3]

Characterization of body size (and the size of mechanical links) is a nontrivial statistical problem because dimensions vary greatly from per-son to person and from population to population. For summary pur-poses, body dimensions are reported typically as means and standard deviations for both males and females within a defined population (e.g., USAF personnel, United States civilians, Japanese civilians, etc.). By assuming that the dimensions follow the Normal (or Gaussian) distribu-tion, body size dimensions can be estimated statistically for various per-centiles of the population of interest. One of the most commonly reported statistics is stature (i.e., standing height). Stature statistics for

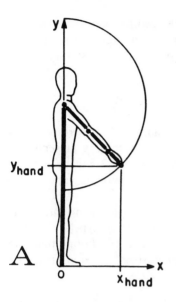

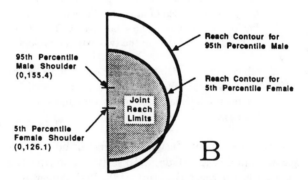

Figure 2. A) Maximum reach limits can be determined by an arc that is located at the shoulder center-of-rotation. B) The "no trunk flexion" reach envelope is determined by simultaneous solution of the large male and small female reach limits.

small (5th percentile), average (50th percentile), and tall (95th percentile) U.S. civilians[20] are summarized in Table IV.

Characterization of the sizes of body links is complicated because link lengths within an individual are not correlated highly. Statistical procedures (some quite complex) have been developed for predicting one link length based on another. One relatively simple procedure has been developed for predicting link lengths based on a person's stature.[21] The method uses the formula:

$$\text{Link length} = K \times \text{Stature}$$

where K is the coefficient, obtained from Figure 3, that corresponds to the link length of interest. The U.S. civilian stature data presented in Table IV and the link length coefficients in Figure 3 can be used to estimate the dimensions of a workstation to accommodate various percentiles of population.

In developing criteria for establishing workstation reach limits, it is essential to select the appropriate anthropometric stereotype(s) for solving a specific design problem. For example, two conditions must be satisfied simultaneously in order to eliminate trunk flexion from the neutral (upright) condition:

1. Objects that are close to the body must be positioned within the reach envelope of a large (95th percentile) male. As shown in Figure 2b, when a worker stands with the arms relaxed at the side of the body, the low reach limit for the large male is more constrained than the low reach limit of the small female. This is due to the difference in hand height between the two extreme population stereotypes.

2. Objects that are displaced horizontally must be positioned within the reach envelope of a small (5th percentile) female. As shown in Figure 2b, the small female has shorter arms and a shorter reach radius than the large male.

A solution to this design problem can be developed using population stature and link length data. To satisfy condition 1, above, it is necessary to describe the reach equation of the 95th percentile male. Geometrically, this can be defined as a circle centered at the shoulder with a radius equal to the length of the arm. Assuming a stature of 186.9 cm and the link length data in Figure 3, the following parameters can be computed:

TABLE IV.   Stature Statistics for U.S. Civilians

Population	Mean (cm)	Std. Dev.	5th %	95th %
Males	175.3	7.1	163.6	186.9
Females	161.5	6.4	151.1	172.2

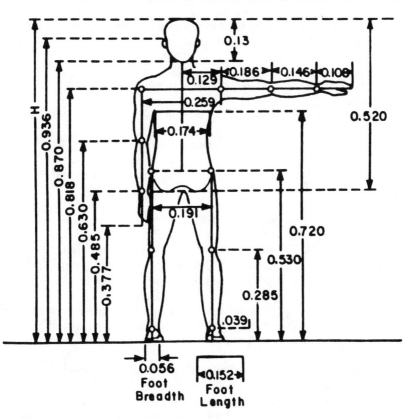

Figure 3. Link lengths of body segments expressed as a proportion of stature.[21]

Shoulder height = 0.818 × 186.9 = 152.9 cm
Upper arm length = 0.186 × 186.9 = 34.8 cm
Forearm length = 0.146 × 186.9 = 27.3 cm
Hand length = 0.108 × 186.9 = 20.2 cm

Reach radius = upper arm + forearm + hand = 82.3 cm

Assuming that shoes increase shoulder height by 2.5 cm, and using the coordinate system of Figure 2a, the center of this circle is located at (0, 155.4), and its Cartesian equation is:

$$X^2 + (Y - 155.4)^2 = 82.3^2 \qquad (1)$$

Similar procedures can be used to describe the reach limits of the small (5th percentile, 163.6 cm) female:

Shoulder height = 0.818 × 151.1 = 123.6 cm
Upper arm length = 0.186 × 151.1 = 28.1 cm
Forearm length = 0.146 × 151.1 = 22.1 cm
Hand length = 0.108 × 151.1 = 16.3 cm

Reach radius = upper arm + forearm + hand = 66.5 cm

Allowing 2.5 cm for shoes, the center of this circle is located at (0, 126.1), and its Cartesian equation is:

$$X^2 + (Y - 126.1)^2 = 66.5^2 \qquad (2)$$

Solving Equations 1 and 2 simultaneously, the intersection occurs at the Cartesian coordinates (61.4, 100.6). These equations and the intersection can be interpreted to develop the following design guidelines:

1. No object should be stored below 73.1 cm ($X = 0$ in equation 1).
2. At heights below 100.6 cm, equation 1 defines maximum reach.
3. At heights above 100.6 cm, equation 2 defines maximum reach.

Caution must be exercised when using maximum reach data. Excessive fatigue and soft tissue injury can result from repeated reaches to the limits of the reach envelope. As a general rule, repetitive reaching should be limited to about one-half of the envelope. Also note that the above recommendations do not consider shoulder problems associated with excessive flexion or abduction. (Shoulder considerations are discussed in the next section.)

For the standard postures described in Figure 1, the neutral position of the trunk allows up to 20 degrees forward flexion. Assuming that 20 degrees of trunk flexion are allowed, and that rotation occurs about the hips, new shoulder coordinates can be computed using link length data and the equations:

$X_{shoulder} = X_{hip}$ + Hip-to-shoulder length × cos 70°
$Y_{shoulder} = Y_{hip}$ + Hip-to-shoulder length × sin 70°

Substituting appropriate values for the 95th percentile male and allowing 2.5 cm for shoes, the new shoulder coordinates are (18.4, 152.1). The corresponding reach equation is:

$$(X - 18.4)^2 + (Y - 152.1)^2 = 82.3^2 \qquad (3)$$

Substituting appropriate values for the 5th percentile female and allowing 2.5 cm for shoes, the new shoulder coordinates are (14.8, 123.5) and the corresponding reach equation is:

$$(X - 14.8)^2 + (Y - 123.5)^2 = 66.5^2 \qquad (4)$$

Solving equations 3 and 4 simultaneously, the intersection occurs at the Cartesian coordinates (72.6, 89.6). These equations and the intersection can be interpreted to develop the following design guidelines to prevent trunk flexion of more than 20 degrees:

1. No object should be stored below 69.8 cm (X = 18.4 in equation 3).
2. At heights below 89.6 cm, equation 3 defines maximum reach.
3. At heights above 89.6 cm, equation 4 defines maximum reach.

By allowing the trunk to flex 20 degrees, the effective reach envelope has been increased slightly in both the vertical and horizontal directions.

Similar procedures could be used to develop reach limit equations that assume limited twisting and lateral bending of the trunk and forearm activities outside of the sagittal plane. It is recommended generally that nonsagittal activities be avoided, however, due to asymmetric loading of spinal tissues.[22]

Guidelines to Prevent Awkward Shoulder Postures

Similar to the trunk, nonneutral postures at the shoulder can be caused by the reach requirements of a task. Shoulder flexion (movement in the sagittal plane) or abduction (movement in the frontal plane) occurs when it is necessary to raise the elbow from its neutral position. (For a person standing with the trunk in a neutral posture as in Figure 2a, the shoulder is considered to be in a neutral position when the upper arm hangs in a relaxed, vertical orientation, parallel to the trunk and the y-axis.) Severely deviated shoulder postures occur when the included angle between the shoulder and the upper arm exceeds 90 degrees, such as when reaching for an object that is positioned too high in the reach envelope.

A general rule of thumb for preventing awkward shoulder posture is:

The lower the reach target, the better the posture.

Therefore, workstation design criteria for preventing awkward shoulder postures should be developed to satisfy the reach limits of the small female. As shown in Figure 2b, the upper reach limits of the small (5th percentile) female are more constrained than those for the large (95th percentile) male. This is due to the lower shoulder height and the shorter reach radius of the small female.

Maximum shoulder height occurs when the trunk is perfectly upright (i.e., when the trunk flexion angle is zero degrees). By keeping the reach target below the maximum shoulder height of the small female, virtually all cases of severe shoulder flexion and abduction can be avoided.

As presented above in the discussion of trunk posture, the shoulder height of the 5th percentile female is 126.1 cm (including a 2.5 cm allowance for shoes). This information can be used to develop the following design guideline:

No object should be stored above 126.1 cm.

Under certain conditions, it is possible for the 5th percentile female to reach above this height without placing the shoulder in a severely deviated posture. To do this, the reach distance between the shoulder and the target must be significantly less than the maximum reach radius (66.5 cm for the small female) and the humerus must be rotated laterally.

Similar to the trunk, recommendations for preventing awkward shoulder posture must be interpreted with extreme caution, particularly when working at the limits of the reach envelope. Repetitive reaches to the limits of the envelope can result in excessive fatigue and/or soft tissue injury.

SUMMARY

The results of the case-referent study suggest that it is possible to use computer-aided posture analysis techniques to identify jobs with an elevated risk for developing back and shoulder pain and disorders. Job redesign, using knowledge of anthropometry and biomechanics can be used to reduce postural risk factors on repetitive jobs.

ACKNOWLEDGMENT

The research presented in this chapter was supported in part through a research contract sponsored by the Ford Motor Company.

REFERENCES

1. Grandjean, E.: *Fitting the Task to the Man*, pp. 41–62. Taylor & Francis, Ltd., London (1980).
2. National Institute for Occupational Safety and Health: *Work Practices Guide for Manual Lifting*. DHHS (NIOSH) Pub. No. 81–122. Cincinnati (1981).
3. Armstrong, T.J.: *Biomechanical Aspects of Upper Extremity Performance and Disorders*. University of Michigan, Department of Environmental and Industrial Health, Ann Arbor (1986).
4. Van Wely, P.: Design and Disease. *Appl. Ergonom. 1*:262–269 (1970).
5. Chaffin, D.B.: Localized Muscle Fatigue – Definition and Measurement. *J. Occup. Med. 15*:346–354 (1973).
6. Andersson, G., R. Ortengren and F. Herberts: Quantitative Electromyographic Studies of Back Muscle Activity Related to Posture and Loading. *Orthop. Clin. North Am. 8*:85–96 (1977).
7. Magora, A.: Investigation of the Relation Between Low Back Pain and Occupation, Part I. *Ind. Med. Surg. 39*:21–37 (November 1970).
8. Magora, A.: Investigation of the Relation Between Low Back Pain and Occupation, Part II. *Ind. Med. Surg. 39*:28–34 (December 1970).
9. Kelsey, J. and R. Hardy: Driving of Motor Vehicles as a Risk Factor for Acute Herniated Lumbar Intervertebral Disk. *Am. J. Epid. 102*:63–73 (1975).
10. Wiker, S.F.: *Effects of Relative Hand Location Upon Movement Time and Fatigue*. Ph.D. dissertation. University of Michigan, Department of Industrial and Operations Engineering, Ann Arbor (1986).
11. Hagberg, M.: Local Shoulder Muscular Strain – Symptoms and Disorders. *J. Human Ergology 11*:99–108 (1982).
12. Bjelle, A., M. Hagberg and G. Michaelsson: Clinical and Ergonomic Factors in Prolonged Shoulder Pain Among Industrial Workers. *Scand. J. Work Env. Health 5*:205–210 (1979).
13. Hagberg, M.: *Prevalence Rates and Odds Ratios of Shoulder and Neck Diseases in Different Occupational Groups*. Unpublished manuscript (1986).
14. Feldman, R., R. Goldman and W. Keyserling: Peripheral Nerve Entrapment Syndromes and Ergonomic Factors. *Am. J. Ind. Med. 4*:661–681 (1983).
15. Keyserling, W.M.: Postural Analysis of the Trunk and Shoulders in Simulated Real Time. *Ergonomics 4*:569–583 (1986).
16. Keyserling, W.M.: A Computer-aided System to Evaluate Postural Stress in the Workplace. *Am. Ind. Hyg. Assoc. J.* (in press, scheduled for October 1986).
17. Karhu, O., P. Kansi and I. Kuorinka: Correcting Working Postures in Industry: A Practical Method for Analysis. *Appl. Ergonom. 8*:199–201 (1977).
18. Kilbom, A., J. Persson and B. Jonsson: *Risk Factors for Work-related Disorders of the Neck and Shoulder – with Special Emphasis on Working*

Postures and Movements. International Symposium on the Ergonomics of Working Posture, Zadar Yugoslavia (1985).

19. Punnett, L., L.J. Fine, W.M. Keyserling, G.D. Herrin and D.B. Chaffin: *Injury and Cumulative Trauma Disorder Surveillance at an Automobile Assembly Plant.* (Work in progress) (1986).

20. National Aeronautics and Space Administration: Anthropometric Source Book Vol. 1, *Anthropometry for Designers*, pp. II.25-II.31. NASA Pub. No. 1024. Washington, DC (1978).

21. Drillis, R. and R. Contini: *Body Segment Parameters.* U.S. Dept. Health, Education and Welfare, Office of Vocational Rehabilitation (1966).

22. Chaffin, D.B. and G. Andersson: *Occupational Biomechanics.* Wiley Interscience, New York (1984).

CHAPTER 3

Biomechanical Strength Models in Industry

DON B. CHAFFIN, Ph.D.

Center for Ergonomics, The University of Michigan, Ann Arbor, Michigan

INTRODUCTION

The act of manually lifting, pushing or pulling an object has been of continual concern to those planning efficient use of a workforce and to those attempting to prevent unnecessary injury and illness in industry. The recent proliferation of industrial robots undoubtedly will decrease the number of workers performing manual material handling jobs, especially if the jobs are highly structured and repetitive. Though estimates are not available as to how fast this displacement of manual labor will occur, it is evident that many manual acts will *not* be automated readily. In particular, automation will be difficult in jobs which are unstructured, especially in the service industries, e.g., building construction, mechanical repair of equipment, baggage and package handling, nurse-patient handling, police protection, and fire fighting, to name a few. A recent report from the National Institute for Occupational Safety and Health stated that approximately one-third of the U.S. workforce is presently required to exert significant strength as part of their jobs.[1]

This same report also presented the following statistics:

- Overexertion was claimed as the cause of lower back pain by over 60% of people suffering from such.

- Disabling overexertion injuries of all types in the U.S. occur to about 500,000 workers per year (which is about 1 in 200 workers each year).

- If the overexertion injuries involve low back pain with significant lost time, less than 1:3 returned to their previous work.

- Overexertion injuries account for about one-fourth of all reported occupational injuries in the U.S., with some industries reporting that over one-half of the total reported injuries are due to overexertion.

- Approximately two-thirds of overexertion injury claims involved lifting loads, and about 20% involved pushing or pulling loads.

Collectively, these observations indicate that manual materials handling activities are now, and will continue to be, prevalent in many industries, and that such acts are associated with either causing or aggravating preexisting musculoskeletal disorders in a large number of workers.

It also became clear from review of pertinent literature that a comprehensive program of control would be necessary.[2] It was proposed that several distinct groups of factors needed to be considered simultaneously in the prevention of musculoskeletal disorders related to manual materials handling.[3] These factors, which define a manual material handling system, were grouped as follows:

- Worker Characteristics
- Work Practices
- Material/Container Characteristics
- Task Characteristics

Often these evoke certain prevention strategies, e.g., worker selection and training, and engineering evaluation and design.

Given the preceding general statements regarding the seriousness and difficulty of resolving the many different human problems resulting from manual materials handling tasks, one must ask:

What can be gained by developing a valid computerized model of worker strengths?

Several different answers can be given. First, consider the more general question: Why model any system? The response is that models are representations which we can understand, even though such representations may require gross simplifications and assumptions. By comparing a model's behavior with the actual behavior of the system, we obtain further insight as to how components of the system function, interact and are coordinated to achieve desired outcomes. Each time a model does not predict a system's behavior correctly, we can rationally change certain parts of the model, thus gaining insight about the complex nature of the real system. It goes without saying that the human biomechanical system is very complex.

In this context one might claim that biomechanical models are strictly academic, serving to enlarge our understanding of musculoskeletal functions. This is certainly one motivation; however, occupational biomechanical models deal with the evaluation of very real situations, i.e., they allow us to determine the maximum allowable magnitude for a load held in various postures, the appropriate size of tools, the least stressful configuration of workplaces and seats, etc. In these situations not only is the human highly variable, but the external loads and postural requirements of different industrial tasks also vary greatly. Because it often is not possible due to time and cost constraints to set up a laboratory simulation of a task and gather adequate performance capacity data from representative volunteers, models are needed. It is often necessary to have normal human performance data available very early in the design of a job so as to consider a variety of alternative job conditions, work methods, and personnel stereotypes. Biomechanical models can sometimes help to rationally interpolate and extrapolate limited musculoskeletal capacity data from different sources to quickly provide specific design guides to complex situations.

Finally, it must be conceded that there are work situations in which a biomechanical model is the only means to predict potentially hazardous loading conditions on certain musculoskeletal components. An example is when one picks up a heavy load. In one posture the load may pose no particular hazard to the low back. In a slightly different posture the combined effects of the load and body weight on the low back exceed limits that most authorities agree are hazardous. A model of the biomechanical properties of a person while performing a specific task can yield such insight.

For these reasons and others, this chapter describes the development of two biomechanical models appropriate to the analysis of manual materials handling situations. The first model represents the static strength capability of workers, while the second model depicts the effects of manual exertions on the low back. Both models are used to solve two common manual material handling tasks.

PLANAR STATIC BIOMECHANICAL MODEL DEVELOPMENT

Biomechanical models begin with the assumption that the whole body can be treated as an articulated linkage system. To illustrate the solution method, consider an anthropometrically average size man holding a load in both hands at about waist height in front of the body. The load is balanced equally between both hands, and the forearms are horizontal. For this example, consider the load to be a 10 kg mass [5 kg in each hand which produces a 49 Newton (N) weight]. The first question is: What rotations moments and forces are acting at the man's elbow due to the external load and the force of gravity acting on the segment mass? By invoking the *first condition of equilibrium*, and with the weight of the forearm and hand assumed to be about 15.8 N for an average man, to maintain the forearm and hand in a static position will require an upward reactive force of 64.8 N at the elbow. This elbow reactive force is created by ligaments and muscle actions at the elbow. In this case the reactive force of 64.8 N is sufficient to keep the forearm and hand from moving in a line (*translation motion*), but it is not able to stop the segment from *rotational motion*.

Because the body segment and load weights act a distance away from the supporting elbow reactive force, they create a *moment*, i.e., a tendency to rotate. The magnitude of a moment is simply the product of a force and the perpendicular distance, i.e., its *lever* or *moment arm* distance, relative to its line of action from the point of rotation. In our example, with the forearm-hand segment held horizontal, its weight has a moment arm from the elbow of 17.2 cm (based on average male anthropometry). Moments, like forces, are vectors and thus direction about a point of rotation as well as magnitude must be considered. The combined moment effects of the two weights, shown in Figure 1, are counteracted by an equal but opposite in direction reactive moment M_E at the elbow; otherwise the segment will rotate. The second condition of equilibrium now can be stated as the sum of moments must equal zero. This yields, when assuming downward forces to be negative:

$$17.2 \text{ cm } (-15.8 \text{ N}) + 35.5 \text{ cm } (-49 \text{ N}) + M_E = 0$$
$$(-271.8 \text{ N cm}) + (-1739.5 \text{ N cm}) + M_E = 0$$

where:

$M_E = 2011.3$ Ncm or about 20 Nm (counterclockwise)

We now have the answer to the question posed earlier regarding the external forces and moments at the elbow during the holding of a 10 kg

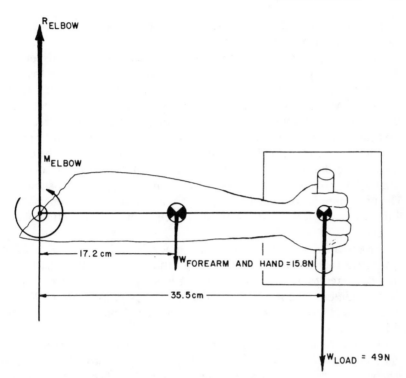

Figure 1.   Free body diagram of forearm and hand in horizontal position holding load.[4]

mass. The reactive moment of a joint is important in that it represents the strength required of specific muscle actions to maintain posture or impart rotational motions.

In the example, if the forearm-hand segment was not horizontal but held at some other angle, the moment at the elbow would be reduced. As the arm is lowered or raised, the moment arms 17.2 cm and 35.5 cm decrease as a function of the cosine of the angle between the forearm and horizontal.

Thus, to estimate the effect of holding a load it is necessary to input two types of data to a strength prediction model:

1. *Task data* which describe the postural angles of the person and any external forces.

2. *Anthropometric data* which describe body segment size and mass characteristics.

Of the two, the task data are most often more significant in determining the strength performance of the population in a given task.

The discussion so far has described a typical static analysis of the external forces acting on one segment of the upper extremity. By treating the body as a kinetic chain, the reactive forces and moments acting at the elbow can be added as vectors to the weight of the upper arm to estimate the effects at the shoulder. Thus, the solution procedure is to first solve the equilibrium equations for the load moments and reactive forces at the joint adjacent to the application of the external load, e.g., at the elbow for our preceding example. Then the resulting values are used to solve the equilibrium conditions for the next adjacent joint, e.g., the shoulder. The procedure is continued in sequence until all the load moments and joint reactive forces are determined at each joint in the kinetic linkage system.

One coplanar, multiple linkage static model is depicted in Figure 2 for symmetric sagittal plane activities while lifting. In this system the forces are considered to act in parallel, thus producing only one force equilibrium condition. The solution procedure was best presented in 1962 by Williams and Lissner[5] for rehabilitation purposes and most recently for industrial tasks.[4]

Since the skeletal muscles respond to load moments, even with simple static models it is possible to gain valuable insight as to what postures required specific muscle groups to be active, and to what relative magnitude each muscle group must contract.

If a kinematic analysis of a person's movement is completed using high speed movies, video, or direct measurement of segment motions, the instantaneous linear accelerations of the mass centers of the segment result.[4] These linear accelerations can be used to directly estimate the dynamic effects, converting the static model to a dynamic model. In most manual materials handling tasks, a good static analysis can provide adequate guidance for job design purposes.

If a dynamic analysis is desired, the means to measure body segment motion parameters is available today, as is the computational capability to resolve the added complexity of dynamic models. Though in many industrial situations static analyses are adequate, dynamic analyses are often needed, e.g., to understand floor slip hazards, climbing, rapid arm motions, etc.[6-8]

Though the two-dimensional coplanar model is very useful in the evaluation of many occupational tasks, in some cases a person will use only one arm when lifting, pushing, or pulling an object while the other arm is used to counterbalance or stabilize the rest of the body. In such a situation the external forces acting on the body must be treated in three

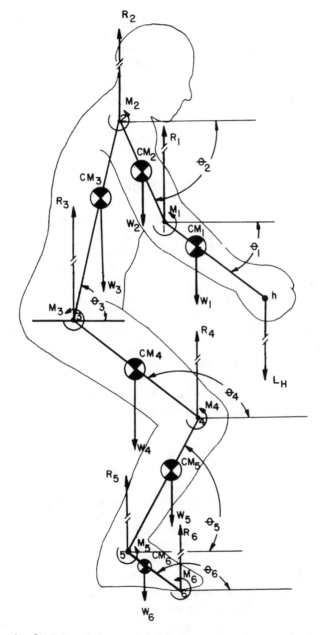

Figure 2.   Six link coplanar parallel static force system for analysis of sagittal plane lifting showing reactive forces and moment at major joints.[4]

dimensions, and the forces are considered to be *non-coplanar*. Basic treatment of the three-dimensional aspects of biomechanical modeling can be found in the test[9] and additional discussion of the topic.[4,10]

Using vector algebra, it is possible to add, subtract and multiply the force and distance values in three dimensions. The computations become quite tedious in a three-dimensional analysis, however. It is for this reason that the solutions must rely on computerized models. Such a model for three-dimensional static strength evaluations of jobs has been developed.[11]

MUSCLE STRENGTH PREDICTION MODELING

The ability to use the muscles to produce moments at each joint appears to be the primary factor limiting many common exertion levels.[12] In essence, this implies that when a person is attempting to lift, push, or pull with a maximal effort, the moments created at each joint due to the application of the load on the hands as well as body weight must be less than or equal to the muscular moment strengths at each joint.

Based on the concept that at each joint there exists a measurable muscle-produced strength moment which cannot be exceeded by the moments created by external loads, biomechanically-based human strength prediction models have been developed.

One of the first static coplanar (sagittal plane) strength prediction models was developed for analysis of load lifting activities.[13] The model can be expressed as a simple set of inequalities at each joint:

$$M_j/L \leq S_j \tag{1}$$

where:

S_j = the muscle-produced moment strengths at each joint (j)
M_j/L = the moments acting at each joint (j) due to external loads (L) on the hands and body segment weights

The M_j/L produce estimates of the moments at each joint for given postures, anthropometry, and external loads. The joint moment strengths, S_j, are obtained by isometric measurements. In this latter regard, it must be recalled that muscle strength moments vary over the range of motion of a joint. Thus, joint angles must be known to predict S_j values and these values have been published.[14-17]

A graphical use of these strength values to predict how much load can be lifted in one hand by average women is shown in Figure 3, assuming

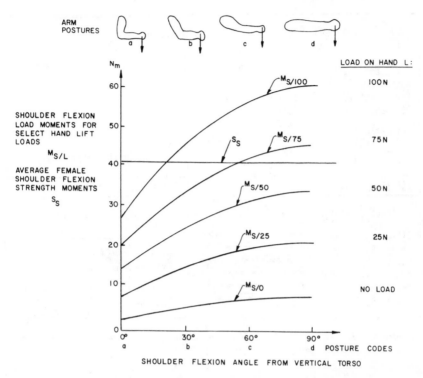

Figure 3.   Shoulder flexion moment required of anthropometrically average women to lift select loads versus predicted average shoulder flexion strength values in the same postures.[4]

the strength limitation is in the shoulder flexion strength moment and not the elbow flexion strength moment. As the load is moved away from the body, the load moments' M_S/L increases while the strength moments' S_S remains relatively constant. Where the M_S/L and S_S values are equal, the average female lifting capability in that arm position is predicted. In other words, when the upper arm is at about 25 degrees, 100 N can be lifted, but when raised to 90 degrees, only 69 N can be held.

By setting the load moments M_j/L equal to the strength S_j at each joint, and rearranging the M_j equations to solve for loads that can be held, it is possible to predict the maximum strength capability for the whole body. In essence, the minimum value of those loads predicted for each muscle strength moment limit is the capability of the whole body exertion.

Because the computations associated with strength modeling are tedi-

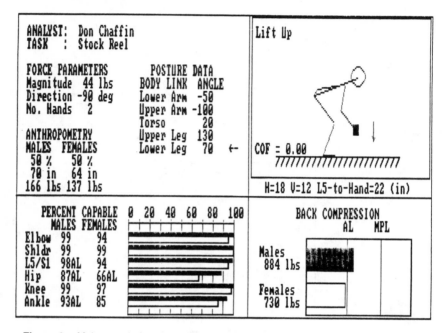

Figure 4. Main screen from The University of Michigan 2D Strength Prediction Program for personal computers.

ous and redundant, computer programs are desirable. The sagittal plane strength model just described was first programmed and used to analyze astronaut lunar exploration activities for NASA in the early 1970s.[18,19] A version of this model is available from the Center for Ergonomics at The University of Michigan for use on personal computers. It is this version that was used to solve the problems discussed later in this chapter. A typical display from this model is shown in Figure 4. The required input values entered from the keyboard are hand load, gross anthropometry, and postural angles. These are shown in the upper left quadrant. The upper right quadrant displays a stick figure of the posture being analyzed. The lower left quandrant is the model's predicted percentage of the population that has the muscle strength at the major joints required by the exertion parameters inputted to the model shown in the upper left quadrant. The lower right quadrant displays the predicted L5/S1 disc compression forces resulting from the exertion. These are graphically compared to the AL (Action Limit) and MPL (Maximum Permissible Limit).[1] The next subsection will discuss the method used to predict the spinal disc compression forces.

Comparison of static muscle strength predictions from these models with whole-body strength exertion data disclose that the model accounts for about 70% of the variation in population strengths for a wide variety of tasks.[20]) The prediction values also tend to be unbiased, i.e., they neither over- or underpredict population strengths, thus allowing the model to be useful in the design and analysis of future manual tasks in industry.

LOW BACK BIOMECHANICAL MODELS

The preceding static model of load lifting has indicated that the moments at the hip joint can become quite large, especially when a load is lifted which cannot be held close to the body. Since the lumbar spine is anatomically close to the hip joints, a similar effect occurs about the joints of the lumbar spine, which in flexion and extension can be considered to be near the center of the spinal discs. In fact, it was proposed that the load moment about the lumbosacral disc (L5/S1) should be used as the basis for setting limits for lifting and carrying loads of various sizes to avoid muscle fatigue and injury in the lumbar extensor (erector spinae) muscle groups.[21]

From a biomechanical perspective, the fact that large moments are created at the lumbar spine when lifting heavy loads raises the question of the nature of the internal forces that must be present to stabilize the spine while incurring such large load moments. A simple static sagittal plane model of the lumbar spine during lifting was proposed.[22] This model assumed that two types of internal forces acted to resist the external load moment. One is the extensor erector spinae muscles that exert their force approximately 5 to 7 cm posterior to the centers of rotation in the spinal discs. The second stabilizing force was assumed to be caused by abdominal pressure acting in front of the spinal column, pushing the upper torso into extension, and thus resisting the load moment acting on the lumbar spine. What resulted from application of this type of model was a realization that large compression forces developed in the spinal column. These acted to compress the discs during a load lifting act. These compression forces were later confirmed in a series of experiments wherein the pressure within the center portion of the discs was measured (by inserting a needle attached to a pressure transducer) on volunteers who performed various lifting maneuvers.[23] Interestingly, separate biomechanical tests of cadaver spinal segments disclosed that the compression forces predicted in the Morris, Lucas and Bressler model of lifting were sufficient to create microfractures of the cartilage endplates between the spinal vertebral bodies and the intervertebral discs.[22,24-26] Further refinement of the model was made to include:[27]

1. Variable anthropometry.
2. Improved spinal geometry for different postures.
3. Abdominal pressure based on hip load moment.

This model is illustrated in Figure 5 and is described completely.[4]

Lifting Variable Loads in Three Different Postures

In this example, consider an anthropometrically average male holding a load of varying magnitude with the load distance from the L5/S1 disc of 30 cm. If the load is incrementally increased in magnitude from no load to over 500 N, the predicted compression force on the L5/S1 disc from the Chaffin model would increase as in Figure 6. The slight nonlinearity in the F_C response is due to the assumed nonlinear abdominal pressure effect.

If the load is moved closer or farther from the torso (H is varied along with the torso and arm postures), the F_C response is greatly affected also. This is particularly informative when the F_C values are compared to the suggested NIOSH Action Limit wherein it is believed some workers would be at risk. This limit is shown in Figure 6 also, along with the Maximum Permissible Limit. What this analysis discloses is that a potential spinal hazard is caused for some workers when they lift a 500 N load close to the body (H = 20 cm) or in lifting a 75 N load farther away from the body (H = 50 cm).

This model also has been used to evaluate varied lifting postures and other industrial tasks.[28]

Three-dimensional Low Back Modeling

The preceding has described a simple coplanar model of lifting which includes a single back muscle force. Additional muscles have been considered in a three-dimensional analysis.[29] An explanation of this model is beyond the scope of this chapter. Suffice it to say that such a model is necessary to analyze the complex forces resulting when one handles a load in other than the sagittal plane.

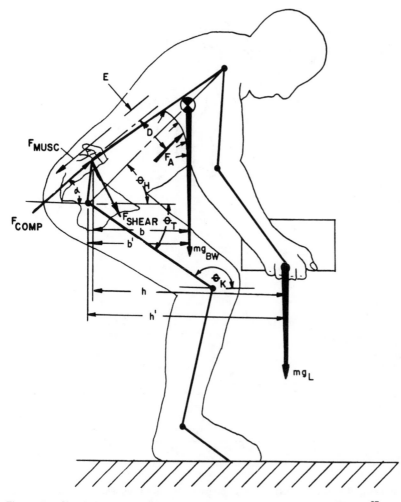

Figure 5.   Simple low back model of lifting for static coplanar lifting analyses.[27]

Case 1: Lifting Stock Roll to Machine Feeder

In this case a roll of stock to be lifted consisted of layers of pliable materials rolled into a cylinder having a 60-cm diameter and weighing 196 N (44 lbs). A worker had to lift the rolls occasionally throughout the day from the floor to two different heights for loading into a stock feeder at waist height and above shoulder height. Because the material was pliable and difficult to grasp, robots were not deemed appropriate.

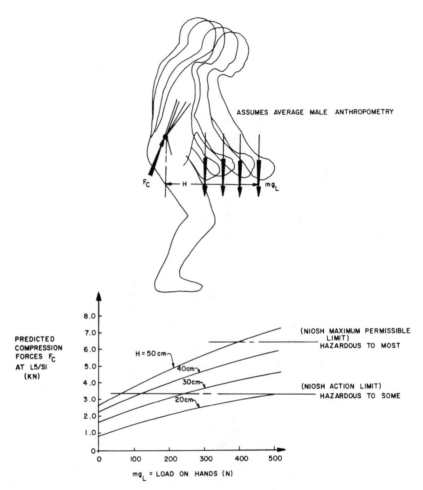

Figure 6. Predicted L5/S1 disc compression forces for varying loads lifted in four different positions from body.

However, some job redesign was deemed to be necessary due to an excessively high number of low back and shoulder complaints.

To evaluate the existing job, videotapes from the side of the workers handling the rolls were obtained. These were viewed in slow motion and stopped at several locations during the lifts. Body angles were measured by protractor from the freeze-frame video and inputted to the PC strength program. Both the percentage of the population (M = male and F = female) having the required muscle strengths at various joints and the spinal compression forces predicted by the model were compared for three postures in the lift.

Figure 7 graphically displays the output from the model for the three postures shown at the top of the figure. What is clear is that the lifting of 196 N from near the floor is particularly hazardous to the low back

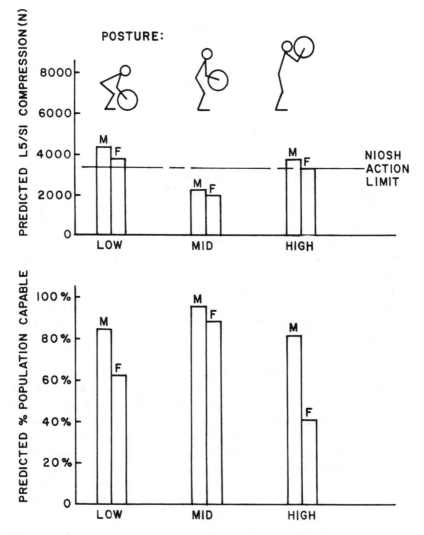

Figure 7. Strength model output from analysis of lifting 196 N (44 lb) roll of stock (60 cm dia) into stock feeder at waist and above shoulder height.

exceeding the NIOSH Action Limit, although 85% of men and 63% of women would have adequate lifting strengths. Also, the above shoulder lifts, although not as hazardous to the back, would be very stressful to the shoulders, with only about 40% of women expected to have sufficient shoulder muscle strengths.

The results of this evaluation confirmed the need to redesign the job to deliver the stock so that it could be grasped and moved without bending over. Also, the stock feeder was redesigned so none of the stock rolls would need to be lifted above shoulder height.

Case 2: Stock Cart Pulling Evaluation

Carts for moving stock from one operation to another are often the source of musculoskeletal injuries. In this particular case, the question was how much load could be placed in the carts under a variety of work conditions. To perform this analysis, a hand-held force-measuring dynamometer was used to measure typical hand forces required to move carts loaded to varying degrees and used under different conditions, e.g., up ramps, over smooth and rough floors, with new and old cart wheels, etc. Once again, videotapes were made of the worker's postures while pulling the carts and the observed postures were inputted to the PC strength model along with the hand forces.

The results of the biomechanical evaluation are graphically depicted in Figure 8. These show that as the hand force required to pull the cart increases beyond about 200 N, the percentage of women capable of exerting such pull forces begins to decrease rapidly.

In addition, it should be noted, that when pushing or pulling on an object, high shear forces are created at the feet that can result in a slip-related injury. The required static coefficient of friction to prevent a foot slip is predicted as part of the latest version of the PC Strength Model and is shown for the cart pulling task in Figure 8. Generally speaking, any task requiring a Coefficient of Friction (COF) above 0.3 must be considered potentially unsafe. As can be seen, when exerting more than 200 N of hand force, an average-sized woman would require about 0.3 COF at the feet. Based on the combined concerns of preventing foot slippage and maximizing cart pulling capability, improved cart maintenance and use policies were implemented.

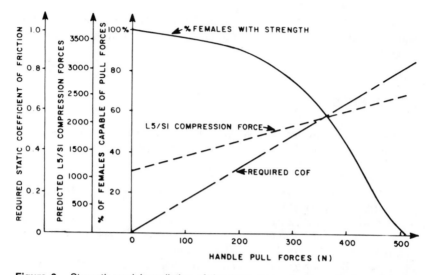

Figure 8. Strength model prediction of the percentage of women having adequate muscle strengths, resulting spinal compression forces, and required COF when pulling with varied hand forces.

SUMMARY AND FUTURE DEVELOPMENTS

The existing static strength models have proven to be very useful in understanding and changing those work conditions that cause occupational musculoskeletal disorders. Any professional concerned with prevention of such disorders needs to be involved in using and contributing to the further development of these methods.

It is clear that we know very little about the mechanical tolerance of various tissues when repeatedly stressed. Bone, muscle, ligament, tendon, and cartilage degeneration is common when frequent stress loading occurs for periods of weeks, months, and even years. The limits to such frequent loadings are not well understood at this time. Biomechanical models will continue to serve a vital role in interpreting and using the limited data that exists as well as indicate the nature of new experiments that must be performed in this regard.

Finally, our existing biomechanical modeling of occupational tasks has been largely static or confined to very simple planar motions. Newer, three-dimensional, high-speed motion sensing and recording systems make it feasible to expand the existing modeling to include more general manual tasks in industry. These new models will be necessarily complex, but with the aid of computer graphics their outputs should be quite useful to engineers and various occupational health and safety professionals concerned with the prevention of mechanical trauma in the workplace.[30]

REFERENCES

1. National Institute for Occupational Safety and Health: *A Work Practices Guide for Manual Lifting*. Technical Report No. 81–122. DHHS, NIOSH, Cincinnati, Ohio (1981).
2. Troup, J.D.B.: Manual Materials Handling—The Medical Problem. *Safety in Manual Materials Handling*, C.G. Drury, Ed. DHHS (NIOSH) Pub. No. 78–185. Cincinnati (1978).
3. Herrin, G.D., D.B. Chaffin and R.S. Mach: *Criteria for Research on the Hazards of Manual Materials-Handling*. Workshop Proceedings on Contract CDC-99-74-118. DHHS, NIOSH, Cincinnati (1974).
4. LeVeau, B.: *Biomechanics of Human Motion*, 2d ed., pp. 150–156. W.B. Saunders, Philadelphia (1977).
5. Chaffin, D.B. and G.B.J. Andersson: *Occupational Biomechanics*. J. Wiley & Sons, New York (1984).
6. Fisher, B.O.: Analysis of Spinal Stresses During Lifting. Unpublished M.S. thesis (Industrial Engineering). The University of Michigan, Ann Arbor (1967).
7. El-Bassoussi, M.M.: A Biomechanical Dynamic Model for Lifting in the Sagittal Plane. Unpublished Ph.D. thesis (Industrial Engineering). Texas Technological University, Lubbock, Texas (1975).
8. Plagenhoef, S.: *Patterns of Human Motion*, pp. 48–55 (1971).
9. Shames, I.H.: *Engineering Mechanics—Statics and Dynamics*, 2d ed. Prentice Hall, Englewood Cliffs, New Jersey (1967).
10. Miller, D.I. and R.C. Nelson: *Biomechanics of Sport*. Henry Kimpton, London (1976).
11. Garg, A. and D.B. Chaffin: A Biomechanic Computerized Simulation of Human Strength. *AIIE Trans. 7(1)*:1–15 (1975).
12. Andersson, G.B.J. and A.B. Schultz: Transmission of Moments Across the Elbow Joint and the Lumbar Spine. *J. Biomech. 12*:747–755 (1979).
13. Chaffin, D.B.: A Computerized Biomechanical Model Development and Use in Studying Gross Body Actions. *J. Biomech. 2*:429–441 (1969).
14. Clarke, H.H.: *Muscle Strength and Endurance in Man*, pp. 39–51. Prentice-Hall, Englewood Cliffs, New Jersey (1966).
15. Schanne, F.A.: A Three-Dimensional Hand Force Capability Model for the Seated Operator. Unpublished Ph.D. thesis (Industrial Engineering). The University of Michigan, Ann Arbor (1972).
16. Burggraaff, J.D.: An Isometric Biomechanical Model for Sagittal Plane Leg Extension. Unpublished M.S. thesis (Industrial Engineering). The University of Michigan, Ann Arbor (1972).

17. Stobbe, T.: The Development of a Practical Strength Testing Program for Industry. Unpublished Ph.D. thesis (Industrial Engineering). The University of Michigan, Ann Arbor (1972).
18. Chaffin, D.B. et al: *Human Strength Simulations for One and Two-Handed Tasks in Zero Gravity*. Biomechanical Division-NASA/MSC, Contract NASA-10973 (1972).
19. Martin, J.B. and D.B. Chaffin: Biomechanical Computerized Simulation of Human Strength in Sagittal Plane Activities. *AIIE Trans. 4(1)*:19–28 (1972).
20. Chaffin, D.B., A. Freivalds and S.R. Evans: On the Validity of an Isometric Biomechanical Model of Worker Strengths. *IIE Transactions* (in press).
21. Tichauer, E.R.: A Pilot Study of the Biomechanics of Lifting in Simulated Industrial Work Situations. *J. Safety Res. 3(3)*:998–1015 (1971).
22. Morris, J.M., D.B. Lucas and B. Bressler: Role of the Trunk in Stability of the Spine. *J. Bone Joint Surg. 43A*:327–351 (1961).
23. Nachemson, A. and G. Elfstrom: Intravital Dynamic Pressure Measurements in Lumbar Disc. *Scand. J. Rehab. Med. Sup. 1*:1–39 (1970).
24. Armstrong, J.R.: *Lumbar Disc Lesions*. Williams and Wilkins, Baltimore (1965).
25. Nachemson, A.: Low-back Pain, Its Etiology and Treatment. *Clin. Med.* 18–24 (1971).
26. Sonoda, T.: Studies of the Strength for Compression, Tension, and Torsion of the Human Vertebral Column. *J. Kyoto Prefect. Med. Univ. 71*:659–702 (1962).
27. Chaffin, D.B.: *On the Validity of Biomechanical Models of the Low-back for Weight Lifting Analysis* (75-WA/BIO-1). American Society of Mechanical Engineers, New York (1975).
28. Park, K.S. and D.B. Chaffin: A Biomechanical Evaluation of Two Methods of Manual Load Lifting. *AIIE Transactions 6(2)*:105–113 (1974).
29. Schultz, A.B. and B.J.G. Andersson: Analysis of Loads on the Lumbar Spine. *Spine 6(1)*:76–82 (1981).
30. Ayoub, M.M. and H.C. Chen: Dynamic Model for Sagittal Lifting. Presented at American Industrial Hygiene Conference, Dallas, Texas (1986).

CHAPTER **4**

Biomechanical Studies in Industry—A Case Study from Cummins Engine Company, Inc.

RANDALL A. RABOURN, MSIE

Center for Ergonomics, The University of Michigan, Ann Arbor, Michigan

INTRODUCTION

This chapter describes the application of biomechanical studies and general ergonomics principles at Cummins Engine Company, Inc. (Cummins), headquartered in Columbus, Indiana. It is not intended to show new research results, but rather to provide a case study of how one manufacturing company and its medical department have implemented and utilized biomechanical studies in an effort to reduce musculoskeletal injuries and provide a safe working environment for employees.

Cummins is the world's largest independent manufacturer of diesel engines for automotive, industrial, and marine applications. Work in the factory is moderately heavy, due to the large size and weight of the engine components assembled and manually handled. Cummins occupational medical services are provided by the Columbus Occupational Health Association (COHA). COHA is a not-for-profit occupational medical organization providing complete outpatient occupational medical care on a fee-for-service basis to its member companies. There are approximately 200 COHA member companies, of which Cummins is by far the largest user of COHA services. All of COHA's staff are Cummins' employees; Cummins is reimbursed for services rendered to and paid by other member companies.

The Cummins occupational biomechanics (ergonomics) activities are conducted by the biomechanics group which is based organizationally within COHA. From 1978 to 1983 this group consisted of one engineer with an ergonomics background and two job analysts; however, currently the group is composed only of the two job analysts. The emphasis of the ergonomics program has evolved since its inception to keep pace with Cummins' needs as Cummins' business environment has changed. The initial emphasis of the program and its projects along with current activities will be discussed.

THE INITIAL BIOMECHANICAL JOB ANALYSIS PROGRAM

The Need for the Program

In the late 1970s, COHA common services provided to Cummins included diagnosing and treating Cummins' employees for occupational injuries and illnesses. COHA would also make recommendations to the Cummins job placement department regarding the type of work these injured employees could perform safely. This was usually done by issuing medical "work restrictions" to workers to reduce their exposure to the work conditions that appeared to be the source of their medical problems. Workers were commonly restricted from exposure to various dermatitis-causing agents and also from various mechanical tasks (e.g., lifting, pushing, and pulling) that might have caused or aggravated their musculoskeletal disorders. The Cummins job placement department would then assign workers reentering the workforce to jobs within their restrictions.

There were several deficiencies with this restricted employee placement system that drew attention from COHA. Workers were often given restrictions to limit the magnitude of a load lifted, pushed, or pulled. This was done to help prevent the occurrence or recurrence of musculoskeletal injuries, especially low back disorders. This index did not take into account such factors as body posture or hand locations, both of which are important in determining the true stressfulness of muscular exertions. The need for a more precise method of classifying muscular exertions was recognized.

Another deficiency was the lack of a uniform system to assess the physical requirements of every job. Consequently, the job placement representative had a difficult task when placing medically restricted employees. It was not uncommon to go through an expensive iterative process of placing and replacing individuals until they arrived at jobs that were consistent with their work restrictions.

One of the primary concerns of COHA that led to the implementation of biomechanical studies was the prevention of low back injuries. This would ideally eliminate employee pain and suffering and the high medical costs often associated with these injuries. Eventually, it would also reduce the need for assigning some medical restrictions. Many of the manual materials handling tasks at Cummins were very strenuous. COHA physicians felt that some workers should not perform these operations even if they had no history of musculoskeletal problems, but there was no mechanism for preventing or reducing exposure to strenuous work tasks that might cause them an overexertion injury.

One potential solution to the muscular exertion problems was to ensure that all workplaces were designed to present little muscular stress so that the vast majority of workers could perform their jobs at a low risk of injury. This would be considered an "engineering" approach to solving the problem. Engineering solutions are usually hardware-oriented and are often expensive to implement in the short-term. They do, however, offer excellent long-term results with little on-going administrative effort and support required.

Another solution was to classify the physical requirements of all jobs systematically and then administratively place workers on jobs according to their individual needs. This latter method could be considered a "clinical" approach and was more suitable to the Cummins organizational structure in which COHA operates. (The COHA ties to placement were much closer than those to engineering departments performing the job design function.) It also provided the framework for placing people according to their strength capability which recently had been shown as a possible way to prevent musculoskeletal injuries in manual materials handling tasks.[1] This latter approach was selected and Cummins embarked on a job analysis program to determine physical requirements. The initial plans for using the job analysis information were:

- To aid the placement of medically restricted workers.
- To assist the physician during patient exams.
- To begin the placement of workers by their strength capabilities to prevent musculoskeletal injuries.

Job Analysis Parameters

Three parameters were chosen to describe the job physical requirements:

- Strength requirements
- Energy expenditure requirements
- General job activities and exposures

The first two were directed toward identifying the manual materials handling factors that might induce musculoskeletal problems and might cause fatigue or certain systemic health problems, respectively. The third was intended to identify general factors that might violate other commonly issued work restrictions.

Job strength requirements were important to know for the placement of workers with musculoskeletal problems and preparation for selective placement by individuals' strength capabilities. In the late 1970s there had been several approaches in describing strength-related issues of manual materials handling, including static and dynamic biomechanical approaches in two- and three-dimensional space and psychophysical modeling.[2-7] A three-dimensional static strength model developed by The University of Michigan was selected and used to quantify the strength requirements of the jobs. Since many jobs are not performed in the sagittal plane or with two hands, this three-dimensional approach was desired. The model's output included the strength required by several different functional muscle groups in terms of the percentile of workers expected to possess enough strength to perform the tasks. The compression force at the L5/S1 disc is also estimated by the model.

Job energy requirements were estimated using metabolic energy cost equations for common work tasks.[8] This information was thought to be important in placing individuals with certain systemic medical problems, such as heart or lung disorders. After surveying approximately 100 jobs, it was discovered that very few jobs required energy expenditure rates over 3 kcal/min. These rates were generally felt to be well within the capability of the workforce. (This was later reinforced by the NIOSH *Work Practices Guide for Manual Lifting*, which indicated that work up to 3.5 kcal/min was considered acceptable.[9]) This portion of the job analysis, therefore, was routinely discontinued and only performed where the analyst felt a moderately high energy expenditure rate might be present.

There were approximately 35 work restrictions which were commonly issued due to employee exposure to specific job factors that might cause or aggravate medical problems such as dermatitis, respiratory allergies or skeletal articulation (joint) disorders. The job analyst used a checklist to identify the general job factors present on each job that would violate these restrictions.

Use of the Job Analysis Information

Over the course of two years and ending in the early 1980s, all manufacturing jobs at Cummins in the Columbus area had been surveyed. This included approximately 1800 different jobs populated by 7000 workers. Information was updated as jobs changed or new jobs were created.

By the time the analyses had been completed, the economic recession in the United States had begun taking its effect upon Cummins. Production rates dropped drastically, entire workshifts were discontinued and, consequently, many workers left the workforce. (The biomechanics group itself had considerable instability. The personnel in the job analyst positions changed several times between 1980 and 1982.) Due to union/ management job placement rules, this mass-movement of employees caused a tremendous amount of shuffling of workers across jobs. The initial plans for using the job analysis data had to be altered. Using the analysis information for the placement of medically restricted workers became even more important than originally thought. This was due to the sheer numbers of employees being moved to different jobs and the fact that between 25 and 30% of the original 7000 workers had medical restrictions. The information pertaining to general work factors was encoded and incorporated into a computer-assisted placement system and used to ease the administration of placing restricted employees. The biomechanics staff also became an important resource to the placement department when there were specific questions or disputes regarding a job's physical requirements during the placement of a particular individual. The biomechanics analysts, as a result of objective and consistent job analyses over time, had gained the trust of both management and the union, and their job findings were respected in addressing these place-ment questions.

The biomechanical strength requirements of specific jobs were available from the analysts to the medical department upon request. As originally intended, this information was used by the physicians during patient examinations to assist in determining the nature and treatment of musculoskeletal injuries and, in some cases, whether or not injuries were occupationally related. This quantitative information about the stresses on specific muscle groups was a valuable supplement to the subjective information offered by the patient.

Placing well employees by strength criteria was never practiced, although much of the preliminary work to begin such a program had been completed. The Cummins' personnel department (and legal representation) was supportive of this program as an extension of the medical job placement system. Isometric strength measuring instrumentation had been procured to measure workers' strength in functional exertions simulating job activities. A battery of functional strength exertions to be tested had been designed by analyzing the biomechanical job analysis data and determining where stressful muscular exertions commonly occurred. In order to implement this strength placement program, it had to be implemented uniformly across all jobs covered in the job placement system to comply with union/management placement rules. It could not be implemented in selected areas only where large strength exertions were common. With the large amount of employee movement due to the economy and the sheer number of employees that would have to be strength tested, it was administratively impractical to conduct such a program.

EXPANDED USE OF THE BIOMECHANICAL STUDIES

Job Redesign Activities

The natural expansion of the use of the biomechanical studies beyond the "clinical" applications eventually took place. In the process of collecting biomechanical job information, the "engineering" application of this information became possible, although this was not a part of the initial plans. Every job had an official work method that was developed by an engineering department. While working with engineering personnel to gather information about specified work methods, informal ties between the biomechanics group and some engineering groups were established. This led to the cooperative redesign of several workplaces which had been found to be biomechanically stressful. Although no formal organizational structure supported it, there were some engineering personnel in local plants who would consult regularly with the biomechanics group to resolve suspected workplace ergonomics problems. Most of the involvement of the biomechanics group with engineering groups was aimed at reducing the risk of back injuries. These types of activities began early in the job analysis project.

Even though the biomechanical studies were not used for employee strength placement, they were used to help identify workplaces in need of redesign. If the biomechanical analysis of jobs indicated that large strength exertions were required, appropriate plant production and safety personnel were notified to help prompt job redesign or work method changes. There were often incidents of overexertion injuries to further support the need for ergonomic improvements.

In addition to manual materials handling problems, there were some incidents of cumulative trauma disorders (CTDs) such as epicondylitis ("tennis elbow"). The biomechanics group was used to help identify high-risk work tasks for CTDs and present potential solutions.

New Job Design Activities

The exposure of the biomechanics group to several plant engineering groups naturally led to some activity in the new job design area. This was not a major portion of this group's work, but "consulting" types of opportunities arose periodically to do such things as evaluate proposed workplace layouts, recommend where materials handling aids and devices were needed, and review proposed new equipment and machine tools for potential ergonomics problems. This activity was not limited to just the local area plants.

CURRENT USE OF BIOMECHANICAL STUDIES AND SERVICES

There are approximately 4000 Cummins production workers today in the Columbus area. Even with this reduced number, it is unlikely that selective placement by strength criteria will be attempted. The downsizing of Cummins workforce has forced many of the once separate work routines to be combined into "interchangeable" work groups. These groups of jobs are then held by groups of workers who might rotate to any of the work routines within the interchangeable group. The intent is to have workers trained to perform any job that is necessary rather than one narrow task. This worker flexibility is expected to lead to an overall improvement in the workforce productivity. Some of the groups contain jobs with quite diverse strength requirements as quantified by biomechanical analyses. In order to ensure that a worker's strength is not mismatched on a job, the most difficult work conditions across all jobs within an interchangeable group would have to be considered the minimum worker strength required to obtain entrance into the group. This approach would be very restrictive.

Interchangeable groups also make it more difficult to place medically restricted workers. Fortunately, the percentage of restricted workers has dropped to 17% of the workforce. The biomechanics group is still very much involved in this process and helps identify jobs within a group which should not be performed by a particular medically restricted worker.

The biomechanics group continues to provide biomechanical job analysis information as needed by physicians during patient examinations, as previously described.

A substantial portion of the Cummins' biomechanics group resources is now devoted to the engineering approach in applying biomechanical studies. New production technology and the need to increase productivity to be competitive in the marketplace have resulted in major revisions to production areas throughout Cummins. Cummins engineering and production staffs are starting to recognize that careful ergonomic design of new workplaces can ultimately enhance productivity and product quality. This should also reduce the incidence of musculoskeletal injuries which in itself improves the overall efficiency of the workforce by reducing medical costs and easing administration of worker placement.

In one large production area currently being remodeled, the biomechanics group is consulted prior to workplace designs being finalized. The design criteria being used for manual materials handling tasks are to provide workplaces that 99% of men and 75% of women would have enough strength to successfully perform, and to keep low back compression forces below 770 pounds. Workplaces are simulated and analyzed by The University of Michigan Biomechanical Model to determine if these criteria are met. These goals correspond to the Action Limit specified in the NIOSH *Work Practices Guide for Manual Lifting*.[9] The NIOSH guide is also being used to supplement the biomechanical analyses to arrive at acceptable lifting frequencies. There is only a limited amount of resources available within the biomechanics group for this type of engineering support, therefore, several engineers have been involved in ergonomic training activities recently in order to become more independent.

SUMMARY

The program of implementing biomechanical studies at Cummins resides in its medical department and began as a means to place workers safely on jobs. The program has survived rather severe economic conditions at Cummins and has taken on the additional dimension of involvement in the engineering job design process. Recently, Cummins has installed a computerized medical surveillance system which presents the opportunity for an on-going epidemiological evaluation of the new job designs.

ACKNOWLEDGMENT

The Cummins Engine Company, Inc. Medical Department was instrumental in the preparation of this manuscript. John Rodway, M.D., Corporate Medical Director, and Don Bundy, Biomechanics Analyst, were particularly helpful in providing information and editorial support.

REFERENCES

1. Chaffin, D.B., G.D. Herrin, W.M. Keyserling and J.A. Foulke: *Pre-Employment Strength Testing in Selecting Workers for Materials Handling Jobs*. DHEW (NIOSH) Pub. No. 77-163 (1977).
2. Ayoub, M.M. and M.M. El-Bassoussi: Dynamic Biomechanical Model for Sagittal Plane Lifting Activities. *Report on International Symposium: Safety in Manual Materials Handling*. DHEW (NIOSH) Pub. No. 78-185 (1978).
3. Chaffin, D.B., G.D. Herrin, W.M. Keyserling and A. Garg: A Method for Evaluating the Biomechanical Stresses Resulting from Manual Materials Handling Jobs. *Am. Ind. Hyg. Assoc. J. 38*:662 (1977).
4. Garg, A. and D.B. Chaffin: A Biomechanical Computerized Simulation of Human Strength. *AIIE Transaction 7(1)*:1–15 (1975).
5. Martin, J.B. and D.B. Chaffin: Biomechanical Computerized Simulation of Human Strength in Sagittal Plane Lifting. *AIIE Transactions 4(1)*:19–28 (1972).
6. Snook, S.H. and V.M. Ciriello: Maximum Weights and Work Loads Acceptable to Female Workers. *J. Occup. Med. 16(8)*:527–534 (1974).
7. Snook, S.H. and V.M. Ciriello: Maximum Weights and Work Loads Acceptable to Male Industrial Workers. *Am. Ind. Hyg. Assoc. J. 31(5)*:571–586 (1970).
8. Garg, A., D.B. Chaffin and G.D. Herrin: Prediction of Metabolic Rates for Manual Materials Handling Jobs. *Am. Ind. Hyg. Assoc. J. 39*:661 (1978).
9. Herrin, G.D., M.M. Ayoub, D.B. Chaffin et al: *Work Practices Guide for Manual Lifting*. DHHS (NIOSH) Pub. No. 81-122 (1981).

CHAPTER 5

Comparison of Different Approaches for the Prevention of Low Back Pain

STOVER H. SNOOK, Ph.D.

Liberty Mutual Insurance Company, Hopkinton, Massachusetts

INTRODUCTION

Low back pain is not a new problem — it was one of the major concerns of Bernardino Ramazzini, the founder of occupational medicine, back in the late 1600s.[1] Low back pain also afflicted the ancient Egyptians of 5000 years ago.[2] Authorities now believe that low back pain existed before humans stood up on their hind legs — and that many four-legged animals currently suffer from this problem.[3]

The specific cause of low back pain is unknown.[3-6] There are many hypotheses, but few objective data. Given the limited knowledge that exists about low back pain, it is doubtful whether the disorder can be prevented totally at the present time. However, there is little doubt that the disability and compensation from low back pain can be reduced substantially to controllable levels.[4,7,8]

Many different preventive techniques have been used in attempting to reduce the problem of low back pain in industry. These techniques can be grouped into three general approaches:

1. Training and education.
2. Job design (ergonomics).
3. Job placement (selection).

The purpose of this chapter is to review the three general approaches and to compare them in their effectiveness in reducing low back pain.

TRAINING AND EDUCATION

Training and education is the oldest and most commonly used approach for reducing low back pain in industry. Training programs have been directed toward workers, management, and practitioners who treat low back pain.

Training the Worker

Safety and/or personnel departments typically have used education and training to instruct employees in proper methods and work procedures. Training in safe lifting has been a part of safety programs in industry for over 50 years. More recent years have seen an increased emphasis on strength and fitness training, and the use of back schools.

Training in Safe Lifting

Several studies have shown that approximately one-half of all compensable low back pain is associated with manual lifting tasks.[9-11] Consequently, there has been a major effort in industry to train workers to lift safely. The original concept of safely lifting an object from the floor required the worker to maintain a straight back, bending the knees to lower the body, and then lifting with the leg muscles. Additional principles of safe lifting were eventually added, e.g., holding the object close to the body; slow, smooth lifting without jerking; turning with the feet instead of twisting the trunk; and the correct positioning of the feet, chin, arms, and hands.[12-15] Unfortunately, there is not always consistency in the content of various safe lifting programs.[16,17]

Two studies have reported 65% and 70% reduction in low back disability as a result of training workers in the principles of safe lifting.[18,19] Unfortunately, these studies were not controlled nor of sufficiently long duration. According to the National Institute for Occupational Safety and Health (NIOSH), the value of training programs in safe lifting is open to question because there have been no controlled studies showing a consequent drop in manual handling accident rate or back injury rate.[20] On the other hand, several studies have reported little or no effect in such training.[11,21,22] Two studies at The University of Michigan investigated the biomechanical aspects of lifting with straight back/bent knees versus lifting with bent back/straight knees. One study concluded that straight back/bent knees should be recommended only for small, compact objects that can be lifted between the knees and close to the body.[23] The other study could find no clear biomechanical rationale for deciding between the two lifting postures.[24]

Strength and Fitness Training

Exercises to increase strength and fitness have been a part of low back pain treatment programs for many years, but only recently have strength and fitness programs been advocated in industry to reduce or prevent the onset of low back pain. Several studies have indicated a positive role for strength and fitness training in reducing the onset of low back pain.[25-27] Three other studies have demonstrated the effects of muscle strengthening exercises in recovering from low back pain.[28-30] However, not all investigations of strength and fitness have demonstrated reductions in low back pain.[31-34]

Although there are conflicting data on the effectiveness of strength and fitness training, the positive evidence appears to outweigh the negative evidence. The most convincing study was conducted by Cady and his associates who used a five-component scale to evaluate the fitness of 1652 firefighters.[25,26] The five components were

1. Endurance work measured (in watts) at the end of twenty minutes of heart rate controlled exercise.

2. Total isometric strength of selected muscle groups.

3. Total of spine flexibility measurements.

4. Diastolic blood pressure during exercise at a heart rate of 160 beats per minute.

5. Heart rate after standardized bicycle exercise.

The firefighters were placed into three groups (most fit, middle fit and least fit) and monitored for compensable low back pain for a period of four years. Approximately 7% of the least fit group experienced low back pain, compared to 3% of the middle fit group, and less than 1% for the most fit group. These investigators were also able to show reduced compensation cost for the most fit individuals. It was concluded that physical fitness and conditioning are preventive of back injuries.

Back Schools

The back school is an attempt to educate the worker in all aspects of back care; it represents a much more comprehensive approach to back care that includes the previous topics of safe lifting, strength and physical fitness. Most back schools include discussions on anatomy and physiology of the lower back, body mechanics, posture, physical fitness, and nutrition. Some back schools will also offer advice on stress management, coping with pain, relaxation, drug use and abuse, first aid and acute care, epidemiology, activities of daily living, and vocational guidance. Job simulation or actual visits to the workplace can also be a part of the back school.

The original concept of the back school was to educate patients who were already suffering (or had recently suffered) from low back pain, i.e., it was a form of treatment. A more recent use of the back school is to educate workers in industry on how to prevent or reduce low back pain. The curriculum is similar, but the students are different in that they may not have experienced low back pain.

There have only been two controlled studies of the effectiveness of a low back school used as a treatment for patients. The first study investigated the effect of the Swedish back school on acute low back pain patients from the Volvo Company in Göteborg, Sweden.[7] Two hundred seventeen patients were randomly assigned to one of three types of treatment: back school, physical therapy, or placebo (treatment with short waves of the lowest possible intensity). The authors concluded that the back school is superior to the placebo and physical therapy in the amount of time required for return to work, and the back school is superior to the placebo in the time required for pain relief. The second study investigated the effect of the Swedish back school on chronic low back patients from an orthopedic center in England.[35] Seventy-eight patients were randomly assigned to the back school or an exercise-only group. Patients in both groups improved in pain and functional disability over the first six weeks. However, patients in the exercise-only group reverted to their original levels of disability at 16 weeks, while back school patients continued to improve.

Preliminary results have been reported for a controlled study of the effectiveness of a low back school as a preventive technique for workers.[36] The program was modeled after the Swedish back school and given to 3424 employees of the Boeing Company in Everett, Washington. There was no significant difference in the incidence of low back pain between the back school students and a similar size control group. The back school also appeared to have little effect on lost work days. The final results of this study have never been published. Other studies have been reported for preventive types of back schools in industry, but they have not been controlled studies. For example, the Southern Pacific Company used the California Back School as a preventive program for 30,000 workers; they report a 22% reduction in low back cases and a 43% reduction in lost work days after two years.[37] PPG Industries used the Atlanta Back School as a preventive program for 2000 workers and report between 70% and 90% reduction in the number of injuries and the cost of injuries after two years.[38] The Spine Education Center in Dallas reports a 40% reduction in lost work days for the year following back schools conducted in eight industries.[39] It is difficult to assess the results of these studies, however, because of the lack of control groups.

Training Management

The use of training and education to prevent or reduce low back pain in industry has been directed almost exclusively toward the worker. Equally important is the training of management. As stated previously, it is doubtful whether low back pain can be totally prevented at the present time. "Secondary prevention" is a technique that is used by management to prevent poor results (i.e., long-term disability) from low back pain that does occur. Poor results are associated with adversary situations, litigation, hospitalization, and lack of follow-up and concern. Management can prevent many of these situations by training foremen, supervisors, and managers in appropriate responses to low back pain.

Data from the Weyerhaeuser Company indicate that workers with back injuries who are off work more than six months have only a 50% possibility of ever returning to productive employment; for more than one year's absence, the possibility is only 25%; for more than two year's absence, the possibility of returning is almost nil.[40] Rosen presents similar statistics.[41] Another study concludes that, with the passage of time following injury, patients increasingly elaborate and exaggerate their symptoms, but are less truly depressed by their predicament.[42] Even if the physical disability remains constant, the patient's psychological posture and the likelihood of returning to work change. These studies emphasize the importance of providing modified, alternative, or part-time work as a means of returning the worker to the job as quickly as possible.[43] Nachemson reviews the evidence suggesting the benefits of early return to work.[44]

Fitzler and Berger describe a program at American Biltrite where management was trained in the positive acceptance of low back pain.[45,46] An atmosphere was created where workers were encouraged to report all episodes of low back pain (even minor episodes) to the company clinic. Immediate and conservative in-house treatment was provided by the company nurse, including worker education. Attempts were made to keep the worker on the job, often with modified duties that were consistent with the worker's condition. If necessary, referrals were made to the company doctor, where treatment and progress were closely monitored. Over a three year period, workers' compensation costs for low back claims were reduced from over $200,000 per year to less than $20,000 per year, a decrease of tenfold. Although this was not a controlled study, the results are certainly impressive.

Training the Practitioner

Company medical personnel should be trained in the benefits of early intervention, conservative treatment, patient follow-up and job placement techniques. Both physicians and nurses should be familiar with recent literature that objectively evaluates various types of treatment for low back pain.[6,47,48] Medical personnel also should be familiar with the physical demands of jobs performed in the company, in order to adequately place injured workers and new employees.

There is little consensus on how low back pain should be diagnosed or treated. Diagnostic criteria and treatment regimens vary greatly among physicians, and may even vary among patients being treated by the same physician.[49] The great variety of treatments and their relative lack of success has frustrated many physicians and patients alike. The most frequently cited source of dissatisfaction with medical care among patients with low back pain is failure to receive an adequate explanation of the problem, resulting in requests for more diagnostic tests.[50]

Wiesel and his associates have offered a standardized approach to the diagnosis and treatment of low back pain.[49] This approach was used by the authors at the Potomac Electric Power Company to monitor the course and treatment for employees with low back pain. If there was any disagreement between the authors (who were orthopedic surgeons) and the treating physician, the latter was contacted for full discussion. Usually, an agreement was reached between the physicians; if not, another physician was consulted for an independent opinion. The number of low back patients decreased 29% the first year and 44% the second year; days lost from work decreased 51% the first year and 89% the second year; and low back surgery dropped 88% the first year and 76% the second year.

JOB DESIGN (ERGONOMICS)

The ergonomic approach of designing the job to fit the capabilities of the worker has received greater attention in recent years. Statistics have been compiled that indicate the relationship of certain job activities and postures to the incidence of compensable low back pain. These activities and postures include manual handling tasks, certain body movements, excessive loads, prolonged sitting, vibration, and falling.

Manual Handling Tasks

More than one-half of all compensable low back pain has been related to the manual handling of objects.[9-11,51] Lifting has been implicated in 37 to 49%° of the cases; pushing, 9 to 16%; pulling, 6 to 9%; and carrying, 5 to 8%. Redesigning jobs to reduce or eliminate the amount of manual handling has been recommended by ergonomists in an attempt to reduce job-related low back pain. Benson reviewed six industrial examples of ergonomic task redesign that resulted in the reduced incidence and cost of compensable low back pain.[52] Working primarily with static loads, Westgaard and Aaras demonstrated a reduction of work-related musculoskeletal illnesses through improved workplace design.[53,54] A 33% reduction in long-term sick leave followed implementation of ergonomic improvements in the workplace.

Body Movements

Excessive bending, twisting, and reaching have been related to the onset of compensable low back pain in industry. Twisting has been reported in 9 to 18% of low back pain; bending in 12 to 14%.[9-11] Twisting the trunk often results from crowded or cramped workplaces where there is not enough room to turn the feet. Bending is necessary when lifting from the floor. Reaching is required when handling bulky objects. Swedish studies have reported that the distance between the object and the body was found to influence the stress on the back much more than the method used to lift.[12]

Excessive Loads

Several studies have related the handling of heavy loads to an increased incidence of low back pain and disability. Hult found almost twice as much low back disability in the heavy occupations as he did in the light occupations.[4] Bergquist-Ullman and Larsson found that manual workers had significantly longer periods of disability during both the initial episode of low back pain and during recurring episodes than office workers.[7] Chaffin and Park concluded that the incidence of low back pain is increased when the lifting load is greater than 35 pounds.[55]

Biomechanical, physiological, psychophysical, and epidemiological criteria have been used for determining excessive loads.[20,56] These critera have been used to develop various methods for evaluating manual handling tasks, e.g., lifting strength rating, job severity index, psychophysical tables, and NIOSH guidelines.[20,55,57,58] Methods based upon biomechanical and psychophysical criteria have been particularly effective in relating low back pain to excessive loads.[11,59-61] Herrin and his associates conclude that the best simple index is the percentage of the population capable of performing the most stressful aspect of a job, based upon either psychophysical strength or isometric strength.[59] Snook used this type of index based upon psychophysical strength and concluded from a study of 191 cases of low back pain that the proper design of manual handling tasks can reduce up to one-third of industrial back injuries.[11]

Additional Risk Factors

Additional risk factors include prolonged sitting, vibration, and falls. Magora's survey of 3316 individuals indicated that too much or too little sitting was related to a higher incidence of low back pain.[62] Nachemson reported that intradiscal pressure during sitting is significantly higher than during standing.[3] Frymoyer and his associates present evidence that implicates vibration as a significant factor in low back pain.[63] Truck drivers, who are exposed to both prolonged sitting and vibration, have a higher incidence of acute herniated lumbar intervertebral discs.[64] Finally, slips and falls have been cited in 7 to 13% of compensable low back pain.[9-11,51] These additional risk factors are important considerations in good job design. Thus far, however, no intervention studies have been reported.

JOB PLACEMENT (SELECTION)

Although job design may be applicable to many manufacturing operations, there are other jobs that are difficult to design and control, e.g., firefighting, police work, and certain construction and delivery operations. These jobs require greater dependence upon preplacement testing and selection of workers. Selection techniques that have been used or suggested for identifying individuals susceptible to future low back pain can be grouped into medical examinations, strength and fitness testing, and job rating programs.

Medical Examinations

The preplacement medical examination has been used in many industries, especially since the enactment of workers' compensation laws. However, there are various opinions in the medical literature regarding the effectiveness of preplacement medical examinations in preventing health and safety problems in industry.[65] Some investigators believe the medical examination should be used only for older workers; others believe it should be used only for hazardous jobs.[65,66] Two studies were unable to demonstrate the effectiveness of preplacement medical examinations in identifying workers who are susceptible to low back pain.[11,67]

Working with 1500 cases of industrial low back pain over a 20-year period, Rowe estimates that, with careful history taking and thorough examination, around seven or eight percent of young individuals prone to future back problems might be identified.[6] The identification rate would be significantly higher in applicants in older age groups where the findings of disease are more frequent and more obvious. Many authorities feel that the medical history is the most important part of the medical examination in identifying workers who are susceptible to future low back pain.[68] Knowing that the worker has had previous low back pain is significant, because the probability of additional episodes of low back pain is four times greater after the initial episode.[69] However, the worker is sometimes reluctant to reveal previous low back pain during a preplacement examination.

Routine X-rays of the lumbar spine have often been part of the preplacement medical examination, although recent evidence indicates that the small yield does not justify the radiation exposure or increased cost.[70,71] Recent advances have been made in measuring the size of the spinal canal by ultrasound. This noninvasive technique was used to show that patients with symptomatic disc lesions had lumbar spinal canals that were significantly more narrow than asymptomatic subjects.[72] A more recent study revealed that coal miners with disabling low back pain also had narrower canals.[73] Other investigators, however, have not yet been able to reproduce these results.[74]

Strength and Fitness Testing

Several studies have demonstrated the relationship between strength/fitness and the incidence of low back pain. In a series of four studies, Chaffin and his associates investigated isometric strength testing as a technique for selecting workers for strenuous jobs.[67,75-78] Workers were tested from various industries (e.g., electronics, steel, aluminum, rubber) and monitored for medical incidents. These studies are consistent in finding that the probability of a musculoskeletal disorder is up to three times greater when job lifting requirements approach or exceed the worker's isometric strength capability.

Several attempts have been made to develop dynamic lifting tests, since dynamic lifting represents a better simulation of the actual lifting task.[79,80] Sophisticated machinery for testing dynamic strength has also been introduced by several manufacturers. Unfortunately, there have been no studies showing the effectiveness of dynamic strength testing as a preplacement technique for reducing the incidence and/or severity of musculoskeletal disorders.

In a Danish study of 449 men and 479 women, Biering-Sorensen was able to show that men who experienced low back pain for the first time had lower isometric endurance of the back muscles when measured up to one year before the episode.[81] In addition, these men also had greater anterior spinal flexion (hypermobility). The results for women were not the same, suggesting a possible sex difference. Biering-Sorensen concludes that good isometric endurance of the back muscles seems to prevent first-time experience of low back pain in men.

Job Rating Programs

Job rating programs are structured attempts to evaluate the job as well as the worker and then obtaining a good match between the two. It represents an extension of not only screening out the inappropriate applicant but finding suitable work for people of varying abilities. Job rating programs began during World War II when military assignments with varying requirements were being filled with millions of new recruits with varying capabilities, and when women, handicapped workers, and older workers began to work in defense factories. Job rating efforts continued after the war when suitable work was being sought for disabled veterans.

One of the pioneers of job rating programs was Hanman, who worked in both Europe and the United States.[82] Koyl developed a job rating program for the Canadian civil service, called GULHEMP (G-general physique, U-upper extremities, L-lower extremities, H-hearing, E-eyesight, M-mentality, P-personality).[83,84] The U.S. National Council on the Aging has advocated the use of GULHEMP for placing older workers on jobs.[83,84] The most recent job rating program has been developed by the County of San Bernardino in California.[85] This program, called the Medical Standards Project, was developed in response to new federal legislation (Civil Rights Act of 1964, Occupational Safety and Health Act of 1970, Vocational Rehabilitation Act of 1973), and increasing disability retirement and workers' compensation claims.

It is not surprising that so much time and effort has gone into the development of job rating programs. These programs appear to provide valuable information regarding worker capabilities and job requirements. It is surprising, however, that not a single study could be found that objectively evaluated the effectiveness of any of the job rating programs in reducing the incidence, severity, or cost of musculoskeletal injuries in the workplace. These programs have good potential, but they remain unproven with respect to injury reduction.

CONCLUSIONS

The reviewed data indicate that primary prevention of low back pain (preventing the onset of symptoms) is best achieved through good ergonomic design of the workplace. Studies have shown that good job design can reduce up to one-third of compensable low back pain. In addition, ergonomics has the advantage of being a more permanent engineering solution to the problem; it reduces the worker's exposure to the risk factors of low back pain and reduces the medical and legal problems of selecting the worker for the job as well as finding replacements for absent workers. Good job design also places less reliance upon the worker's willingness to follow established training procedures, such as lifting properly.

Strength testing is an effective selection technique, but should only be used for jobs that are difficult to design or control. Strength testing can also be used on a temporary basis until the job is redesigned. Strength testing should never be used as a substitute for good job design.

Training the worker in strength and fitness also appears to be effective in preventing the onset of low back pain symptoms. Although fitness is difficult to enforce, management can encourage worker participation by supplying facilities and training programs.

Secondary prevention (preventing long-term disability and high cost after low back pain has occurred) is best achieved through training programs. Specifically, management should be trained in appropriate responses to low back pain, practitioners should be trained in effective treatment, and patients should be sent to back school to learn their responsibilities in the recovery process.

Ergonomics also plays an important role in secondary prevention. Not only can good job design reduce the probability of initial and recurring episodes, it will also allow the worker with moderate symptoms to stay on the job longer and permit the disabled worker to return to the job sooner.

There is no simple solution to the problem of low back pain. No single preventive approach will solve the problem: all approaches are necessary for the control of low back pain. However, prevention programs should emphasize those approaches that objective studies have shown to be most effective. Although knowledge about low back pain is limited, enough is already known to control the problem adequately. Instead of waiting for a major medical breakthrough to occur, emphasis should be placed on applying the knowledge that is already available.

REFERENCES

1. Mastromatteo, E.: From Ramazzini to Occupational Health Today From an International Perspective. *J. Occup. Med. 17*:289–294 (1975).
2. Finneson, B.E.: *Dr. Finneson on Low Back Pain*. G.P. Putnam's Sons, New York (1975).
3. Nachemson, A.L.: Towards a Better Understanding of Low Back Pain: A Review of the Mechanics of the Lumbar Disc. *Rheum. Rehab. 14*:129–143 (1975).
4. Hult, L.: Cervical, Dorsal and Lumbar Spine Syndromes. *Acta Orthop. Scand. Suppl. No. 17* (1954).
5. Jayson, M.I.V.: Back Pain: Some New Approaches. *Med. J. Austral. 1*:513–516 (1979).
6. Rowe, M.L.: *Backache at Work*. Perinton Press, Fairport, New York (1983).
7. Bergquist-Ullman, M. and U. Larsson: Acute Low Back Pain in Industry. *Acta Orthop. Scand. Suppl. No. 170* (1977).
8. Cust, G., J.C.G. Pearson and A. Mair: The Prevalence of Low Back Pain in Nurses. *Int. Nurs. Rev. 19*:169–179 (1972).
9. Cady, L.D., D.P. Bischoff, E.R. O'Connell et al: Letters to the Editor: Authors' Response. *J. Occup. Med. 21*:720–725 (1979).
10. Snook, S.H., R.A. Campanelli and R.J. Ford: *A Study of Back Injuries at Pratt and Whitney Aircraft*. Liberty Mutual Insurance Company, Research Center, Hopkinton, MA (1980).
11. Snook, S.H., R.A. Campanelli and J.W. Hart: A Study of Three Preventive Approaches to Low Back Injury. *J. Occup. Med. 20*:478–481 (1978).

12. Andersson, G.B.J., R. Ortengren and A. Nachemson: Quantitative Studies of Back Loads in Lifting. *Spine 1*:178–185 (1976).

13. Anderson, T.M.: Human Kinetics in Strain Prevention. *Brit. J. Occup. Safety 8*:248–250 (1970).

14. Himbury, S.: *Kinetic Methods of Manual Handling in Industry.* Occupational Safety and Health Series No. 10. International Labour Office, Geneva (1967).

15. National Safety Council: Human Kinetics . . . and Lifting. *Nat. Safety News*, pp. 44–47 (June 1971).

16. Hall, H.W., Sr.: "Clean" vs "Dirty" Leaning, an Academic Subject for Youth. *ASSE J.*:20–25 (October 1973).

17. Ring, L.: *Facts on Backs—A Simplified Approach to Back Injury Prevention and Control.* Institute Press, Loganville, Georgia (1981).

18. Glover, J.R.: Prevention of Back Pain. *The Lumbar Spine and Back Pain.* M. Jayson, Ed. Grune and Stratton, New York (1976).

19. Miller, R.L.: Bend Your Knees! *Nat. Safety News*, pp. 57–58 (May 1977).

20. U.S. Department of Health and Human Services: *Work Practices Guide for Manual Lifting.* DHHS (NIOSH) Pub. No. 81–122 (March 1981).

21. Brown, J.R.: *Lifting as an Industrial Hazard.* Labour Safety Council of Ontario, Ontario Department of Labour, Toronto (1971).

22. Dehlin, O., B. Hedenrud and J. Horal: Back Symptoms in Nursing Aides in a Geriatric Hospital. *Scand. J. Rehabil. Med. 8*:47–53 (1976).

23. Park, K.S. and D.B. Chaffin: A Biomechanical Evaluation of Two Methods of Manual Load Lifting. *AIIE Trans. 6*:105–113 (1974).

24. Garg, A. and G.O. Herrin: Stoop or Squat: A Biomechanical and Metabolic Evaluation. *AIIE Trans. 11*:293–302 (1979).

25. Cady, L.D., D.P. Bischoff, E.R. O'Connell et al: Strength and Fitness and Subsequent Back Injuries in Firefighters. *J. Occup. Med. 21*:269–272 (1979).

26. Cady, L.D., P.C. Thomas and R.J. Karwasky: Program for Increasing Health and Physical Fitness of Firefighters. *J. Occup. Med. 27*:110–114 (1985).

27. Rowe, M.L.: Low Back Pain in Industry. A Position Chapter. *J. Occup. Med. 11*:161–169 (1969).

28. Kraus, H., W. Nagler and A. Melleby: Evaluation of an Exercise Program for Low Back Pain. *Am. Fam. Physician 28*:153–158 (1983).

29. Kendall, P.H. and J.M. Jenkins: Exercises for Backache: A Double-blind Controlled Trial. *Physiotherapy 54*:154–157 (1968).

30. Lindstrom, A. and M. Zachrisson: Physical Therapy on Low Back Pain and Sciatica: An Attempt at Evaluation. *Scan. J. Rehabil. Med. 2*:37–42 (1970).

31. Pedersen, O.F., R. Petersen and E.S. Staffeldt: Back Pain and Isometric Back Muscle Strength of Workers in a Danish Factory. *Scan. J. Rehabil. Med. 7*:125–128 (1975).

32. Gyntelberg, F.: One Year Incidence of Low Back Pain Among Male Residents of Copenhagen Aged 40–59. *Dan. Med. Bull. 21*:30–36 (1974).

33. Berkson, M., A. Schultz, A. Nachemson and G. Andersson: Voluntary

Strengths of Male Adults with Acute Low Back Syndromes. *Clin. Orthop.* *129*:84–95 (1977).

34. Nachemson, A.L. and M. Lindh: Measurement of Abdominal and Back Muscle Strength With and Without Low Back Pain. *Scand. J. Rehabil. Med.* *1*:60–65 (1969).

35. Klaber Moffett, J.A., S.M. Chase, I. Portek and J.R. Ennis: A Controlled, Prospective Study to Evaluate the Effectiveness of a Back School in the Relief of Chronic Low Back Pain. *Spine 11*:120–122 (1986).

36. Nordin, M., V. Frankel and D.M. Spengler: *A Preventive Back Care Program for Industry* (Abstract). International Lumbar Spine Society Meeting, Paris, May 17–20 1981.

37. Pilcher, O.J.: Personal Correspondence (February 9, 1979).

38. Johnson, C.D.: Safety Forum. *Ind. Safety Prod. News* (June 21, 1981).

39. Melton, B.: Back Injury Prevention Means Education. *Occup. Health Safety*, pp. 20–23 (July 1983).

40. McGill, C.M.: Industrial Back Problems: A Control Program. *J. Occup. Med. 10*:174–178 (1968).

41. Rosen, N.B.: Treating the Many Facets of Pain. *Business & Health*, pp. 7–10 (May 1986)

42. Beals, R.K. and N.W. Hickman: Industrial Injuries of the Back and Extremities. *J. Bone Joint Surg. (Am.) 51A*:1593–1611 (1972).

43. Derebery, V.J. and W.H. Tullis: Delayed Recovery in the Patient with a Work Compensable Injury. *J. Occup. Med. 25*:829–835 (1983).

44. Nachemson, A.L.: Work for All. *Clin. Orth. 179*:77–85 (1983).

45. Fitzler, S.L. and R.A. Berger: Attitudinal Change: The Chelsea Back Program. *Occup. Health Safety*, pp. 24–26 (February 1982).

46. Fitzler, S.L. and R.A. Berger: Chelsea Back Program: One Year Later. *Occup. Health Safety*, pp. 52–54 (July 1983).

47. Deyo, R.A.: Conservative Therapy for Low Back Pain — Distinguishing Useful from Useless Therapy. *JAMA 250*:1057–1062 (1983).

48. Quinet, R.J. and N.M. Hadler: Diagnosis and Treatment of Backache. *Arth. Rheum. 8*:261–287 (1979).

49. Wiesel, S.W., H.L. Feffer and R.H. Rothman: Industrial Low Back Pain: A Prospective Evaluation of a Standardized Diagnostic and Treatment Protocol. *Spine 9*:199–203 (1984).

50. Deyo, R.A. and A.K. Diehl: Patient Satisfaction with Medical Care for Low-back Pain. *Spine 11*:28–30 (1986).

51. Bigos, S.J., D.M. Spengler, N.A. Martin et al: Back Injuries in Industry: A Retrospective Study. II. Injury Factors. *Spine 11*:246–251 (1986).

52. Benson, J.D.: Control of Low Back Pain in Industry Through Ergonomic Redesign of Manual Materials Handling Tasks. *Trends in Ergonomics/Human Factors III*, W. Karwowski, Ed. Amsterdam, North Holland (1986).

53. Westgaard, R.H. and A. Aaras: Postural Muscle Strain as a Causal Factor in the Development of Musculoskeletal Illnesses. *Appl. Ergo. 15*:162–174 (1984).

54. Westgaard, R.H. and A. Aaras: The Effect of Improved Workplace Design on the Development of Work-related Musculoskeletal Illnesses. *Appl. Ergo.* *16*:91–97 (1985).

55. Chaffin, D.B. and K.S. Park: A Longitudinal Study of Low-back Pain as Associated with Occupational Weight Lifting Factors. *Am. Ind. Hyg. Assoc. J.* *34*:513–525 (1973).

56. Snook, S.H.: Workloads. *Proceedings of an International Symposium on Low Back Pain and Industrial and Social Disablement.* Back Pain Association, London (October 7, 1982).

57. Ayoub M.M., N.J. Bethea, S. Deivanyagam et al: *Determination and Modeling of Lifting Capacity.* Final Report. DHEW/NIOSH Grant No. 5 R01 OH D0545–02 (1978).

58. Snook, S.H.: The Design of Manual Handling Tasks. *Ergonomics* *21*:963–985 (1978).

59. Herrin, G.D., M. Jaraiedi and C.K. Anderson: Prediction of Overexertion Injuries Using Biomechanical and Psychophysical Models. *Am. Ind. Hyg. Assoc. J.* *47*:322–330 (1986).

60. Liles, D.H., S. Deivanyagam, M.M. Ayoub and P. Mahajan: A Job Severity Index for the Evaluation and Control of Lifting Injury. *Human Factors* *26*:683–693 (1984).

61. Liles, D.H. and P. Mahajan: Using NIOSH Lifting Guide Decreases Risks of Back Injuries. *Occup. Health Safety*, pp. 57–60 (February 1985).

62. Magora, A.: Investigation of the Relation Between Low Back Pain and Occupation. *Ind. Med.* *41*:5–9 (1972).

63. Frymoyer, J.W., M.H. Pope, J.H. Clements et al: Risk Factors in Low Back Pain. *J. Bone Joint Surg.* *65-A*:213–218 (1983).

64. Kelsey, J.L.: An Epidemiological Study of Acute Herniated Lumbar Intervertebral Discs. *Rheumatol. Rehabil.* *14*:144–159 (1975).

65. Schussler, T., A.J. Kaminer, V.L. Power and I.H. Pomper: The Preplacement Examination. *J. Occup. Med.* *17*:254–257 (1975).

66. Alexander, R.W., A.S. Maida and R.J. Walker: The Validity of Preemployment Medical Evaluations. *J. Occup. Med.* *17*:687–692 (1975).

67. Chaffin, D.B., G.D. Herrin and W.M. Keyserling: *Pre-employment Strength Testing in Selecting Workers for Materials Handling Jobs.* U.S. Dept. Health Education and Welfare (NIOSH) CDC-99-74-62 (1976).

68. Lipson, S.J.: Adult Low Back Pain. *Current Concepts.* The Upjohn Co. (1982).

69. Dillane, J.B., J. Fry and G. Kalton: Acute Back Syndrome – A Study from General Practice. *Brit. Med. J.* *2*:82–84 (July 1966).

70. Montgomery, C.H.: Preemployment Back X-rays. *J. Occup. Med.* *18*:495–498 (1976).

71. American Occupational Medical Association: Guidelines for Use of Routine X-ray Examinations in Occupational Medicine. *J. Occup. Med.* *21*:500–502 (1979).

72. Porter, R.W., C. Hibbert and P. Wellman: Backache and the Lumbar Spinal Canal. *Spine 5*:99–105 (1980).

73. Macdonald, E.B., R. Porter, C. Hibbert and J. Hart: The Relationship Between Spinal Canal Diameter and Back Pain in Coal Miners. *Occup. Med. 26*:23–28 (1984).

74. Feffer, H.L.: Editorial Commentary: Ultrasonography of the Spine. *J. Occup. Med. 26*:28 (1984).

75. Chaffin, D.B.: Human Strength Capability and Low-back Pain. *J. Occup. Med. 16*:248–254 (1974).

76. Chaffin, D.B., G.D. Herrin and W.M. Keyserling: Preemployment Strength Testing: An Updated Position. *J. Occup. Med. 20*:403–408 (1978).

77. Keyserling, W.M., G.D. Herrin and D.B. Chaffin: Isometric Strength Testing as a Means of Controlling Medical Incidents on Strenuous Jobs. *J. Occup Med. 22*:332–336 (1980).

78. Keyserling, W.M., G.D. Herrin, D.B. Chaffin et al: Establishing an Industrial Strength Testing Program. *Am. Ind. Hyg. Assoc. J. 41*:730–736 (1980).

79. Kamon, E., D. Kiser and J.L. Pytel: Dynamic and Static Lifting Capacity and Muscular Strength of Steelmill Workers. *Am. Ind. Hyg. Assoc. J. 43*:853–857 (1982).

80. Kroemer, K.H.E.: Testing Individual Capability to Lift Material: Repeatability of a Dynamic Test Compared with Static Testing. *J. Safety Research 16*:1–7 (1985).

81. Biering-Sorensen, F.: Physical Measurements as Risk Indicators for Low-back Trouble Over a One-year Period. *Spine 9*:106–119 (1984).

82. Hanman, B.: *Physical Capacities and Job Placement.* Nordisk Rotogravyr, Stockholm (1951).

83. Koyl, L.F., M. Hackney and R.D. Holloway: *Employing the Older Worker: Matching the Employee to the Job.* The National Council on The Aging, Washington (1974).

84. Nelson, N.: *Technical Training Guide for Physical Demands Analysis.* The National Council on The Aging, Washington (1984).

85. Nylander, S.W. and G. Carmeau: *Medical Standards Project Final Report,* 3rd ed. County of San Bernardino, CA (1984).

CHAPTER 6

Evaluation and Design of Jobs for Control of Cumulative Trauma Disorders

THOMAS J. ARMSTRONG, B.S.E., M.P.H., Ph.D., and
YAIR LIFSHITZ, M.S.

Center for Ergonomics, The University of Michigan, Ann Arbor, Michigan

INTRODUCTION

Industrial Hygiene is concerned with the recognition, evaluation and control of biological, chemical, physical, and ergonomic stresses. There are generally accepted procedures for evaluating and controlling most biological, chemical, and physical stresses. Such is not the case for many of the ergonomic stresses that can cause, precipitate, or aggravate upper extremity cumulative trauma disorders. Ergonomic problems most often are identified from medical records and insurance claims after they already have occurred.[1] The relationship between many ergonomic problems and their causes simply is not understood well enough to predict with certainty the risk of a problem occurring in a given work situation. Furthermore, it is not always possible to determine if a proposed control measure will indeed remedy a problem. Therefore, control measures should be regarded as hypotheses until their effectiveness has been verified experimentally. This chapter addresses evaluation and design of jobs for generating hypotheses for control of cumulative trauma disorders. Evaluation of the hypotheses are discussed by Silverstein.[2]

Ideally, epidemiological procedures can be used to isolate the specific disorders and their associated causes, such as carpal tunnel syndrome associated with the use of a certain type of tool or tendinitis in the wrist associated with a certain task; however, it is seldom possible to isolate the problem and causes so accurately and precisely. Under most circumstances it is only possible to show an excess morbidity of cumulative trauma disorders in a given production area of a plant. Usually, a production area contains a variety of jobs and tools, and it is necessary to evaluate all of the jobs in the affected area for recognized risk factors and corresponding causes. Once the likely risk factors have been identified, control measures and ways of evaluating them can be proposed.

IDENTIFICATION OF RISK FACTORS

Cumulative trauma disorders are similar to diseases caused by chemical contaminants in that a dose-response relationship is hypothesized to exist between the agent and the disorder. While it is possible to define a chemical dose, a mechanical dose is not as well defined. Commonly cited risk factors (repetitiveness, forcefulness, mechanical stresses, posture, vibration) all contribute to tissue trauma. Although it is not possible to define and measure the stress dose itself, it is possible to identify and reduce or eliminate the factors associated with tissue trauma. The following describes procedures that can be used to analyze jobs for these factors. Procedures vary from simple to complex; as might be expected, the amount of information obtained about the job and risk factors is related to the complexity of the analysis. The availability of microcomputers and suitable software shows great promise for decreasing the complexity and increasing the quality of these analyses.

All job analysis schemes are based on some kind of checklist in which risk factors are either recorded or rated. They vary in the level of detail with which the job is scrutinized. At the simplest level, the analyst watches one or more workers perform the job and checks off the risk factors as they are observed.

A checklist suitable for analyzing jobs in "real time" is shown in Figure 1. It consists of a list of the recognized risk factors — repetitiveness, forcefulness, mechanical stresses, postures, and physical stresses.[3] Along with each factor is a sublist of specific job attributes to look for, e.g., forceful exertions often are associated with lifting, holding, assembling, use of tools, gloves, and pinching. Mechanical stresses often are associated with gripping tools, or resting the arms on the sharp edges of a workbench, desk, or machine. Posture must be considered for each joint: the hand, wrist, elbow, and shoulder.[4] Stressful postures result from the use of tools, materials, or controls at certain locations with respect to the worker.

The checklist, shown in Figure 1, is intended to be very general; it can be made specific for given types of jobs or industries. For example, to

Plant: Area:
Job: Worker:

1. Repetitiveness:

    a. A single task, motion, or posture is performed more than 50% of the time
    b. The production standard exceeds 900 units per shift

2. Forcefulness: Are forceful exertions required to:

    a. lift
    b. hold
    c. assemble
    d. use tool
    e. use gloves
    f. pinching

3. Mechanical stresses on the fingers, hands, wrists, elbows, arms:

    a. tools
    b. controls
    c. parts
    d. machines
    e. workbench
    f. keyboards
    g. desks

4. Posture: wrist deviation
             wrist flexion
             wrist hyperextension
             elbow flexion
             extreme supination
             extreme pronation
             shoulder: elbows raised more than 30°
             elbows behind torso

    a. reaching for: control, material, tool
    b. using: control, material, tool
    c. assembling

5. Physical stresses:

    Vibration:

    a. hand-held power tools
    b. bench-mounted power tools
    c. impact tools
    d. vehicle controls

    Skin temperatures below 70°F

    a. cold ambient air
    b. gripping cold tools or parts
    c. cold air exhaust

Figure 1.   Checklist for identification of upper extremity cumulative trauma disorder
              risk factors.

tailor the checklist for office settings, types of jobs might be listed to indicate repetitiveness; a word processing operator and a receptionist might represent the extremes of high and low repetitiveness. Sharp edges on desks and keyboards might be used to indicate mechanical stresses. It probably would not be necessary to investigate vibration exposure in the office. A checklist developed at one site should not be used at a second site until an on-site inspection of jobs that encompass the various extremes of repetitiveness, forcefulness, mechanical stress, posture, and vibration has been performed.

The use of the checklist discussed thus far has been qualitative. It is possible to make such a checklist quantitative by making additional checks every time an item is observed. It then is possible to calculate the total number of stressful exertions.[5] Further refinements can be achieved by including dimensions or other quantitative information about the workplace or by annotating factors as necessary. Simple "yes-no" checklists are most useful for "walkthrough" surveys where it is desirable to determine if there is a possible problem and a need for further analysis or for epidemiological studies.

A checklist used by Lifshitz and Armstrong[6] to evaluate job designs for control of cumulative trauma disorders is shown in Figure 2. The analyst scores the job by checking only those items that apply to that situation. It would not be necessary to score item 3.2, "Can the tool be used without flexion or extension of the wrist?" if hand tools are not used for the job. The final score then is calculated as the fraction or percentage of the responses scored as yes. A score of 0% implies maximum job stress; a score of 100% implies minimum job stress. A correlation ($r^2 = 0.75$) was found between the total checklist scores and the incidence of cumulative trauma disorders among workers in a surgical products plant. In a more recent study, the checklist was applied to 30 jobs populated by 652 workers reported Armstrong et al.[3] A correlation of 0.82 between overall checklist scores and the prevalence of cumulative trauma disorders was found. Although the overall scores are useful for epidemiological purposes, it usually is desirable to calculate a total subscore for each category of risk factors. The subscores indicate where the attention should be focused to control the problem.

The job analysis can be made more systematic if the work objective, station and method are formally described. The first step is to state the objective of the job. Examples might include hem pant legs, remove fat from ham, install connector on cable. The second step is to describe the sequence of work elements that the worker must perform to accomplish the objective.[3] Formal procedures for describing work elements based on

1. Physical Stress:

    1.1 Can the job be done without contact of fingers or wrist with sharp edges?
    1.2 Is the tool operating without vibration?
    1.3 Are the worker's hands exposed to temperature > 70°?
    1.4 Can the job be done without using gloves?

2. Force

    2.1 Does the job require less than 10 pounds of force?
    2.2 Can the job be done without using finger pinch grip?

3. Posture

    3.1 Can the job be done without flexion or extension of the wrist?
    3.2 Can the tool be used without flexion or extension of the wrist?
    3.3 Can the job be done without deviating the wrist side to side (ulnar or radial deviation)?
    3.4 Can the tool be used without ulnar or radial deviation of the wrist?
    3.5 Can the worker be seated while performing the job?
    3.6 Can the job be done without "clothes wringing" motion?

4. Workstation hardware

    4.1 Can the orientation of the work surface be adjusted?
    4.2 Can the height of the work surface be adjusted?
    4.3 Can the location of the tool be adjusted?

5. Repetitiveness

    5.1 Is the cycle time above 30 seconds?

6. Tool design

    6.1 Can the thumb and finger slightly overlap around a closed grip?
    6.2 Is the span of the tool's handle between 5 and 8 cm?
    6.3 Is the handle of the tool made from material other than metal?
    6.4 Is the weight of the tool below ten (10) lbs?
    6.5 Is the tool suspended?

Figure 2. Checklist for analysis of upper extremity cumulative trauma disorder risk factors.[6]

the work of Gilbreth are described by Barnes[7] and by Niebel.[8] The elements required to hem pant legs are listed in Figure 3.

The level of specificity of these steps varies from general to detailed descriptions of the movements and exertions of each hand. A simplified analysis of hemming pant legs is shown in Figure 4. The required work equipment includes a 30-inch high sewing table with sharp formica edges, a Brand X sewing machine, and a chair. The checklist is applied by examining each work element, the equipment, and parts for items on the

Left Hand	Right hand
Reach to a trouser	Reach to a trouser
Grasp a trouser	Grasp a trouser
Position trouser	Position trouser
Hold trouser hold ⎫	Hold trouser hold ⎫
Move trouser ⎬ × 4	Move trouser ⎬ × 4
Position trouser ⎭	Position trouser ⎭
Move trouser aside	Move trouser aside
Release trouser	Release trouser

Problems:

1. Forceful exertions are required to hold the trouser while sewing.
2. Ulnar deviation of the wrist while sewing.
3. Wrist extension while performing the operation.

Recommendations:

1. Change the orientation of the sewing table so that the worker can perform the job without ulnar deviation of the wrist or wrist extension.
2. Provide an adjustable chair to the operator.

Figure 3.   Elemental analysis of Hem Pant Leg.

Simplified Work Elements

Get	trouser
Hold	trouser
Return	trouser

Figure 4.   Simplified analysis of Hem Pant Leg.

checklist. The results of applying the checklist to the "hem pant leg" job are shown in Figure 5. The overall score is 30%. Scores of 0% imply problems in the force, workstation hardware, and repetitiveness categories. The results of applying the checklist do not necessarily differ when the elemental analysis is performed than when it is not. The elemental analysis will increase the likelihood of finding a problem and generally is recommended.

A further refinement of the system entails quantitatively measuring each of the factors. For example, wrist posture can be measured and plotted as described by Armstrong et al.[9] Wrist postures and hand forces for the "hem pant leg" job are shown plotted in Figure 6. The job now can be scored in terms of the percentage of time spent in a stressful

Checklist Score for Hem Pant Leg

CTD Factor	%
Physical stress	100
Force	0
Posture	50
Workstation hardware	0
Repetitiveness	0
Tool design	N/A
Overall score	30

Figure 5. Checklist for analysis of upper extremity cumulative trauma disorder risk factors proposed by Lifshitz and Armstrong[6] applied to Hem Pant Leg.

posture, or as the number of stressful exertions per unit of time. These measures are very useful for epidemiological studies and for comparing one job design with another. Unfortunately, there is not a quick and accurate way to continuously measure upper extremity posture. Most investigators rely on a frame by frame visual analysis of film or video tapes.[5,9] Recent developments in electrical goniometers and microcomputer systems show great promise for reducing the equipment and labor costs of quantitative posture and force measurements. Only a few of these are adaptable to in-plant kinds of studies. One such system is shown in Figure 7.[3] The time and equipment overhead of such systems presently are too great for them to be practical job survey tools.

To determine the overall risk of cumulative trauma disorders or the risk associated with parts of the job, it is necessary to compare force, repetitiveness, and posture data with predetermined action limits. Unfortunately, such action limits are not known with nearly the accuracy with which it is possible to measure force, repetitiveness, and posture. The major uses of detailed force and posture analyses in the immediate future are for comparisons of alternative work equipment and epidemiological studies.

Another way of analyzing jobs is on paper. For example, instead of timing the job with a stop watch to determine its repetitiveness, the average cycle time can be computed from the published work standard, from production records, or from payroll records. If the job is not yet in production, this information sometimes can be determined from predetermined time standards or standard time data. A methods analysis can be used to determine both the type and number of exertions required to complete each work unit. The number of similar movements should be

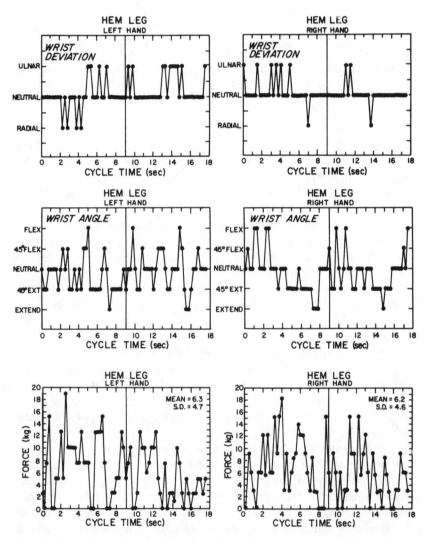

Figure 6. Wrist postures and hand forces demonstrated in two cycles of Hem Pant Leg.

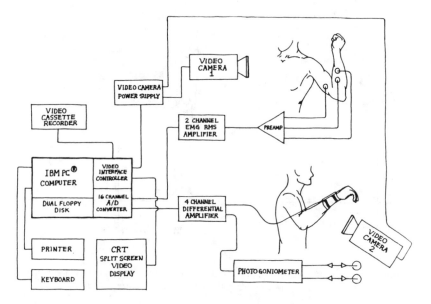

Figure 7. A computerized system for in-plant collection of posture and force data.[11]

multiplied by the number of work units to determine the overall repetitiveness.

The types of exertion can be used to determine where contact with controls, tools, parts, and equipment might produce mechanical stresses on the body. Information about the controls, tools, parts, and equipment often can be obtained from catalogues, engineering drawings, or by examining similar systems which are in operation.

Information about the location and orientation of controls, tools, parts, and equipment can be used to determine the work posture required for workers of given size.[3] Figure 8a shows how an anthropometric drawing board mannikin can be used to determine that a small female would have to lean against the edge of the table to reach a palm button located 30 inches from the worker at a height of 48 inches. By comparing Figure 8a with the checklist in Figure 1, use of the palm button is related to postural stress in the shoulder, contact stresses from the edge of the bench, and the palm button. Also, there may be an excessive force requirement associated with the palm button. Pencil and paper analyses also are useful for design of interventions and new jobs. Figure 8b shows how relocating the palm buttons 20 inches horizontally and 40 inches vertically effectively reduces the postural stress on the shoulder. The use

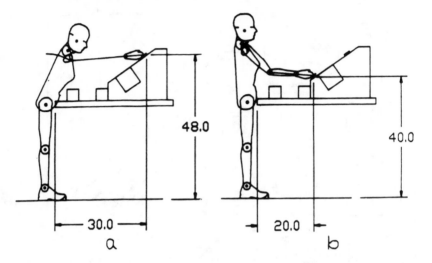

Figure 8.   Use of computer-aided drafting program to evaluate two control locations a and b for someone with 5th percentile female stature.

of anthropometric mannikins in workstations has been greatly enhanced by the availability of computer-aided design hardware and software. Figures 8a and 8b were constructed on a microcomputer-based system described by Armstrong et al.[3] Such files can be plotted or stored on magnetic disks for later editing to evaluate the ergonomics consequences and possible job changes. While the anthropometric mannikins and computers are helpful, they are not essential. Figure 9 shows how simple stick figures, based on body proportions from Drillis and Contini,[10] can be created to evaluate the posture of tall and short workers using pistol and inline powered screwdrivers on various work surfaces.[11]

CONTROL MEASURES

There always are ways of eliminating the causes of cumulative trauma disorders. The problems becomes one of economy, i.e., of finding solutions that are not too expensive to implement or that adversely affect production. While it frequently is argued that safety and health improvements lead to increased returns by preventing losses and improving labor relations and productivity, this is, in fact, hard to prove, especially to a manager who does not understand ergonomics and cannot take a long view of things. It is very difficult to develop general principles for convincing management to make ergonomic job improvements. Once man-

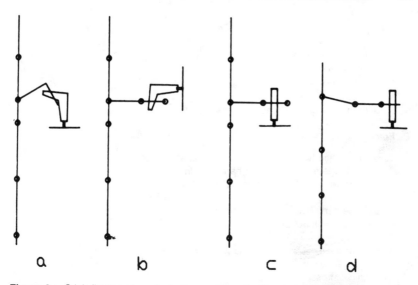

a   b   c   d

Figure 9. Stick figures to evaluate the posture of tall and short workers using pistol and inline powered screwdrivers on various work surfaces.[11]

agement has made a commitment, each organization must develop its own criteria for determining the cost-effectiveness of control measures.[12,13]

The general principles for designing control measures for intervening in cumulative trauma disorders have been reviewed in other papers.[3,14-16] They are briefly summarized in Figure 10.

Although the proposed interventions may seen very logical and likely to result in an improved checklist score, they should be considered experimental until they have been evaluated. Formal schemes for evaluation interventions for cumulative trauma disorders are discussed by Silverstein.[2]

SUMMARY

Reported risk factors of cumulative trauma disorders include forcefulness, repetitiveness, mechanical stress, certain postures, and physical stresses. Checklists of risk factors are useful tools for identifying possible causes of cumulative trauma disorders. They can be tailored to focus on job attributes specific to each industry. They also can be made quantitative by computing the fraction of affirmative responses. They can be further enhanced by analyzing work content and quantitative measure-

A. Repetitiveness

   1. Use mechanical aids
   2. Enlarge work content
   3. Rotate workers
   4. Increase allowance
   5. Spread work uniformly across workshift

B. Force

   1. Decrease the weight of tools, containers, and parts
   2. Increase the friction between handles and the hand
   3. Optimize size and shape of handles
   4. Select gloves to minimize effects on performance
   5. Balance hand-held tools and containers
   6. Use torque control devices
   7. Optimize pace
   8. Mechanical assists

C. Mechanical stress

   1. Enlarge corners and edges
   2. Pads and cushions
   3. Materials

D. Posture

   1. Locate work properly
   2. Orient work properly
   3. Select tool design for workstation

E. Vibration

   1. Select tools with minimum vibration
   2. Select process to minimize surface and edge finishing
   3. Mechanical assists
   4. Use isolation for tools that operate above resonance point
   5. Provide damping for tools that operate at resonance point
   6. Adjust tool speed to avoid resonance

Figure 10.   Common interventions for control of cumulative trauma disorders.

ment of joint position and force. Such measurements are useful for evaluating alternative job designs and for epidemiological studies, but probably are not warranted for routine survey work. Once the causes have been identified, interventions can be proposed. Such interventions, however, should be regarded as experimental until their effectiveness can be substantiated through controlled field studies.

REFERENCES

1. Fine, L., B. Silverstein, T. Armstrong et al.: Detection of Cumulative Trauma Disorders of Upper Extremities in the Workplace. *J. Occup. Med.* 28:674–678 (1986).

2. Silverstein, B.: Evaluation of Interventions for Control of Cumulative Trauma Disorder. Presented at Symposium on Ergonomic Interventions to Prevent Musculoskeletal Injuries in Industry, Denver, CO, October 9–10 1986. (See Chapter 7 in this book).

3. Armstrong, T., R. Radwin, D. Hanson and K. Kennedy: Repetitive Trauma Disorder, Job Evaluation and Design. *Human Factors 28*:325–336 (1986).

4. Armstrong, T.: Ergonomics and Cumulative Trauma Disorders. *Hand Clinics 2*:553–565 (1986).

5. Drury, C. and J. Wick: Ergonomic Application in the Shoe Industry. *Proceedings of the 1984 International Conference on Occupational Ergonomics,* pp. 489–493. Toronto (1984).

6. Lifshitz, Y. and T. Armstrong: A Design Checklist for Control and Prediction of Cumulative Trauma Disorders in Hand Intensive Manual Jobs. *Proceedings of the 30th Annual Meeting of Human Factor,* pp. 837–841 (1986).

7. Barnes, R.: *Motion and Time Study, Design, and Measurement of Work.* John Wiley & Sons, New York (1972).

8. Niebel, B.: *Motion and Time Study,* 7th ed. Richard D. Irwin, Inc., Homewood, IL (1982).

9. Armstrong, T., J. Foulke, B. Joseph and S. Goldstein: Investigation of Cumulative Trauma Disorders in a Poultry Processing Plant. *Am. Ind. Hyg. Assoc. J. 43*:103–116 (1982).

10. Drillis, R. and R. Contini: *Body Segment Parameters BP 174–94.* Tech. Rep. No. 1166.03. School of Engineering and Science, New York University, New York, NY (1966).

11. Armstrong, T.: Upper Extremity Posture; Definition, Measurement and Control. *The Ergonomics of Working Postures, Models Methods and Cases,* pp. 59–73. N. Corlett, J. Wilson and I. Manenica, Eds. Taylor and Francis (1986).

12. McKenzie, F., J. Storment, P. Van Hook and T.J. Armstrong: *Am. Ind. Hyg. J. 46*:674–678 (1985).

13. Joseph, B.S.: A Participative Ergonomics Control Program in a U.S. Automotive Plant: Evaluation and Implication. Unpublished Ph.D. dissertation. The University of Michigan, Ann Arbor (1986).

14. Tichauer, E.: Some Aspects of Stress on the Forearm and Hand in Industry. *J. Occup. Med. 8*:63–71 (1966).

15. Tichauer, E.: Biomechanics Sustains Occupational Safety and Health. *Industrial Engineering,* pp. 46–56 (1976).

16. VanBergeijk, E.: Selection of Power Tools and Mechanical Assists for Control of Occupational Hand and Wrist Injuries. Presented at the Symposium on Ergonomic Interventions to Prevent Musculoskeletal Injuries in Industry, October 9–10, 1986, Denver, CO (See Chapter 12 in this book).

CHAPTER 7

Evaluation of Interventions for Control of Cumulative Trauma Disorders

BARBARA A. SILVERSTEIN, M.P.H., Ph.D.

School of Public Health, The University of Michigan, Ann Arbor, Michigan

INTRODUCTION

Cumulative trauma disorders (CTDs) include chronic soft tissue problems of the musculoskeletal and peripheral nerve systems. Occupational risk factors associated with upper extremity CTDs include repetitive or forceful exertions particularly in combination with sustained or awkward postures, mechanical stress, vibration, gloves, or cold temperatures. Most would agree that the major components of a CTD control program are

1. Identification of developing health problems.
2. Identification of job risk factors.
3. Implementation of control measures.
4. Evaluation of the effectiveness of the controls.

While most in-plant ergonomic programs would agree that evaluation is an important component of any program, very few have used systematic ways of evaluating whether the stated objectives have been met. These stated objectives of most in-plant ergonomic programs include:

1. Reduce medical visits.
2. Reduce cost of injuries.
3. Increase product quality.
4. Improve employee job satisfaction.
5. Increase productivity.

TYPES OF INTERVENTIONS AND EVALUATIONS

These objectives are not always compatible. Nor are they mutually exclusive necessarily. The latter three objectives often are viewed as natural by-products of the first two objectives. The extent to which this might be true depends on the type of intervention used to address a particular problem in a given situation within the context of external and technology constraints. Control strategies have been discussed in detail elsewhere. Briefly, they fall under five broad headings:

1. Engineering modifications of workstations, tools or parts.
2. Administrative controls such as employee selection and restriction.
3. Organization of work such as enlargement, work groups, rotation, flowline reorganization, rotation.
4. Training in work methods or ergonomic awareness.
5. Personal protective equipment such as pads, gloves, sleeves.

Many use an "anecdotal approach" to evaluation rather than documenting changes in risk factors and subsequent changes in health outcomes. The anecdotal approach can be characterized by "Let's go look at a job" analysis of risk factors with no systematic analysis or documentation of findings and a sporadic follow-up evaluation of success including "no more complaints" or "asked the operator." While it is necessary to involve the operator at all stages of the intervention process to increase the probability of acceptance, this is not sufficient. This approach does not lend itself to generalizing interventions to similar types of jobs. As long as this is true, there will continue to be more individual fires igniting than an ergonomics program can extinguish successfully. This default approach to evaluation is used in many in-plant programs because accurate recordkeeping is often the first victim discarded while fighting ergonomic fires. Currently, the effectiveness of these programs is being accepted, in large part, on faith. When the day of reckoning comes, without documentation the entire ergonomic program may go up in the same smoke. From a public health perspective, preventing high-risk jobs from entering the workplace is less expensive and more effective than curing (retrofitting) existing jobs.

Making the Connection

In order to determine whether an ergonomic intervention is successful in controlling CTDs, we have to determine whether the exposure is associated with the health outcome(s) of interest. First, did the exposure occur prior to the health outcome or CTD? If there is increased exposure (duration or intensity), is there increased effect? If there is less exposure (the intervention), does a decrease in incidence or prevalence follow? If so, are there any other factors that explain these changes?

In order to answer these questions, the same valid and reliable measures of exposure and outcome must be used either to compare groups with different levels of exposure or the same group before and after the intervention. Similarly, baseline data on cost of CTDs (in-plant and personal medical visits and treatments, restrictions, lost time, retraining, compensation claims), quality (scrap and repair rates), and productivity (standards, labor variance, downtime, output volume, material and machine utilization, etc.) must be collected for future comparisons if achievement of these objectives is to be evaluated as part of ergonomic program effectiveness. While this seems obvious, it is often very difficult to do.[1]

METHODOLOGICAL ISSUES

Evaluations of interventions in occupational health studies are notoriously difficult for a variety of methodological and practical reasons. These include small numbers, difficulties in measuring exposure and health outcomes, resource and time constraints, types of interventions implemented, and a variety of external factors.

Sample Size

If the difference in proportion of CTDs between high-risk and low-risk groups is great, then relatively small numbers in each group may be adequate to detect statistically significant results. For example, as part of a prevalence study in an electronics plant, we identified a statistically significant 17-fold increased risk of wrist tenosynovitis among workers in high force–high repetitive jobs compared to low force–low repetitive jobs (Table I). On the other hand, when we used 33 handpackers in a dental floss plant as their own controls in evaluating the preliminary impact of an exercise program on neck shoulder symptoms, a twofold difference was observed, but not statistically significant (Table II). The number of persons required in a comparison of groups with different risks depends on the proportion of CTDs in the baseline or comparison group, the power and certainty required (Tables III and IV).

One way of getting around small numbers problems is to develop and

TABLE I. Wrist Tenosynovitis on History and Physical Examination among Telephone Manufacturer Employees Based on Job Characteristics

	High Repetitive High Force	Low Repetitive Low Force	Total
Disease	9 (a)	0 (b)	9
No Disease	15 (c)	23 (d)	38
Total	24 (e)	23 (f)	47

Odds Ratio (a × d)/(b × c) = 28.81
(Fisher Exact P = 0.00096)
Prevalence Ratio (a/e)/(b/f) = 17.64
(p < .005)

TABLE II. Neck Shoulder Cumulative Trauma Disorder Symptoms among Handpackers Before and After Five Months of Exercise

Neck Shoulder CTDs	1986 yes	1986 no
1985 yes	16	2
1985 no	4	11

Odds Ratio = 0.5
(0.03, 4.33)

McNemar's Test (paired chi square)

focus on a "risk factor database" rather than specific jobs or departments. This information can also be used in placement of restricted workers, thereby decreasing lost time cases and costs. Of course, this assumes that the relationship between risk factors and CTDs is understood.

When employees serve as their own controls in intervention studies, observations are not independent. McNemar's paired chi square test is appropriate for categorical analysis.[3] With continuous exposure (risk factor scores) or outcome variables (severity index), repeated measures analysis of variance or covariance are useful statistical techniques.[1]

Health Outcomes

There are often limitations in traditional plant measures of health outcomes.[4] These include:

1. Limited exposure data.
2. Reporting biases, including distance to medical department, type of problem, trust of medical department.

TABLE III.   Sample Size Requirements to Determine Simple Differences in Proportions with 90% Power and 95% Certainty

Group 1 Rate	Group 2 Rate	# per Group
5%	10%	621
10%	15%	957
10%	20%	286
10%	30%	92
20%	25%	1504
20%	40%	118
20%	60%	34

From Fleiss.[2]

TABLE IV.   Sample Size Requirements for Paired Case Control Studies with 90% Power and 95% Certainty

Baseline Rate	Difference	# of Pairs
5%	5% less	72
10%	5% less	300
20%	10% less	136
30%	15% less	81

From Schlesselman.[3]

3. Inconsistent recordkeeping.
4. Inconsistent diagnostic criteria.
5. Time lag (OK—exposure—symptom—physical findings—interventions—physical findings—symptoms—OK).

Risk Factors

There are a variety of limitations which affect our ability to assess job risk factors accurately. These include:

1. Employee variability (anthropometry influences postural risk factors).
2. Task variability even on the "same job."
3. Competing risk factors (force, repetitiveness).
4. Lack of knowledge about how risk factors interact or how much is too much.
5. Lack of resources to analyze every job and every worker performing the job.

6. Job changes (unrelated to ergonomic programs) which may change the risk factors or eliminate the job.
7. Employees may face multiple exposures on the same job or by rotating through different jobs. What is an appropriate time-weighted average for multiple risk factors?

Additionally, employees may have a variety of personal risk factors which may increase their probability of developing CTDs. These include a variety of chronic diseases including many autoimmune and metabolic diseases, age, acute traumatic injuries, aggravating hobbies, or outside activities.[5] The relationship between these personal and occupational factors is not well understood.

External Factors

External factors that affect the organization may have a greater impact on medical visits and risk factors than specific ergonomic interventions on specific jobs. For example, these might include:

1. Changes in the economy and labor market have a greater impact on absenteeism and job turnover than most internal changes.[6,7]
2. Changes in medical benefits and workers' compensation may alter which avenue employees will choose for reporting CTDs.
3. Changes in production technology and product lines may eliminate high risk jobs or leave only survivors on remaining jobs. Alternatively, older workers at increased personal risk may be placed on unaccustomed jobs or have increased intensity of exposure on remaining jobs.

Several examples are illustrative of these difficulties.

Example 1

A midwestern gauze and tape plant was concerned about the incidence of CTDs in the plant (particularly carpal tunnel syndrome) and initiated an ergonomics program in 1981. Plant medical records were reviewed to target problem jobs and with the intention of establishing baseline incidence rates for future comparisons. A variety of jobs were analyzed and recommendations were made by both corporate and University of Michigan ergonomists. A number of these recommendations were implemented including those which decreased awkward postures, mechanical stress, and forcefulness.

The plantwide incidence of CTDs (based on plant medical records) was

TABLE V.   Plantwide Incidence Rates of Upper Extremity CTDs and Events in a
Midwestern Gauze and Tape Plant, 1980–1985

Year	Hours	CTD # (rate)
1980	1,363,070	35 (5.1)
1981	1,154,257	29 (5.0)
Plan Move to New Plant 30 Miles		
1982	739,957	27 (7.3)
Move, Elim. Depts.		
1983	No data	No data
1984 New MD	306,282	14 (9.1)
1985	245,894	12 (9.8)

TABLE VI.   Plantwide Incidence Rates of Carpal Tunnel Syndrome and Events in a
Midwestern Gauze and Tape Plant, 1980–1985

Year	Hours	CTD # (rate)
1980	1,363,070	9 (1.3)
1981	1,154,257	6 (1.0)
Plan Move to New Plant 30 Miles		
1982	739,957	5 (1.4)
Move, Elim. Depts.		
1983	No data	No data
1984 New MD	306,282	5 (3.3)
1985	245,894	2 (1.6)

5.1 per 200,000 work hours in 1980 and 9.8 per 200,000 work hours in
1985 (Table V). The plantwide incidence for carpal tunnel syndrome did
not change between 1980 (1.3/200,000 hours) and 1985 (1.6/200,000
hours) (Table VI). Based on this information, this ergonomic program
does not appear to be very effective in reducing medical incidence of
CTDs.

This example illustrates a number of the problems encountered in
attempting to evaluate the effectiveness of the interventions and program. These include:

1. Small numbers. The plant population was reduced from 682 in 1980
   to 123 in 1985. As the number of cases and number at risk decrease,
   rates become more unstable. Incident rates for specific jobs or even
   departments (in which there are very different risk factors) are even
   more unstable. In this plant population, it would be very difficult to
   obtain statistically significant differences either by comparing the
   differences in proportion of CTDs for those pre/post intervention
   studies (Table IV).

2. Measures of health outcome. In the above example, plant medical records were relatively good. Even with good reporting forms, a change in plant physicians may have resulted in inconsistent record-keeping and inconsistent diagnostic criteria. There may be differential reporting to plant medical by employees for a variety of reasons. Additionally, an increase in reporting of CTDs may be an indication of program success if it represents early reporting and decrease in severity over time.

3. Measures of risk factors. Observation of all workers performing the same jobs was not possible. Systematic review of risk factors after implementation of interventions by local plant personnel was not possible. Although some risk factors may have been reduced, they may not have been the most important ones but rather the easiest ones to change. A number of suggested controls may not have been feasible or justifiable to plant personnel in the face of moving these problem jobs to other plants.

4. External factors. As plans for downsizing the plant operations, elimination of not only specific jobs but whole departments, and moving the plant progressed, a variety of poorly documented factors were introduced. Who were the employees left? Not only were they most likely older (personal risk factor) but had more seniority (increased duration of exposure) than those laid off. Concern about job security and the future may have influenced reporting of symptoms. This could have had two contradictory effects. On the one hand, concerned employees may have overreported in order to establish their future compensation claims. On the other hand, those with enough seniority to remain on the job may have been either survivors or worried that reporting of symptoms may result in layoff.

Example 2

In conjunction with a study of upper extremity CTDs among women sewing machine operators in an automotive upholstery plant,[8] it was noted on physical examination that a number of women who used scissors on their jobs had evidence of mechanical stress on the dorsal surfaces of the fingers that came in contact with the traditional scissor handle bales (blisters, calluses, discomfort). In order to evaluate the effectiveness of alternative scissors designs in reducing mechanical stress and discomfort, a localized postural discomfort survey adapted from the work of Corlett and Bishop[9] was used. Contour mapping of the location of discomfort in the scissors hand, similar to that used by Karlqvist,[10] was also used. Initially, operators from each of three "scissors exposed" groups were provided with six different commercially available and four laboratory-fabricated scissors which they ranked in order of preference. The three scissors designs chosen by the operators had self-opening springs (one manufactured by Stirex and two lab-fabricated types) and no mechanical stresses on the dorsal fingers.[11] Each group of ten randomly selected operators were to use their own scissors for a week and then each of the other scissors for a week. Postural discomfort surveys were conducted (scoring from 1 = no discomfort to 10 = intolerable discomfort) four times during the course of the Monday of the trial and once during midshift Friday of the same week for each week of the testing. While there was significantly less discomfort reported with the Stirex scissors than the original scissors, the lab-fabricated scissors resulted in more discomfort. This discomfort was transferred from the dorsal surfaces of the fingers to the palmar surfaces due to excess force required to close the fabricated scissors. The discomfort was great enough that operators did not use these scissors for more than several days at most. Of additional interest was the finding of significantly decreased discomfort after two weeks vacation from any scissors use.[11]

The sensitivity of the postural discomfort survey and contour mapping of discomfort suggests that these are useful surrogate measures for musculoskeletal disease which requires more resources to identify and more lag time between decrease in exposure and decrease in physical findings. The use of postural discomfort as a surrogate measure is advocated strongly by Webb[12] and has been found to be promising in providing relatively rapid feedback which can be used to fine tune interventions in our own studies. We are in the process of determining whether these surveys are predictive of CTDs and can be used as an effective early warning system in in-plant control programs.

Example 3

Westgaard and Aaras[13,14] describe the effect of improved workplace design on the incidence of musculoskeletal disorders in a Norwegian telephone exchange cable manufacturing plant between 1967 when the plant opened and 1982. According to the authors, by 1974, musculoskeletal-related sick leaves and turnovers were increasing dramatically. Measures of health effect included medical diagnoses collected at the local health authority for all sick leaves lasting more than three days. In 1979, all workers were questioned about the intensity and location of pain (past and present). Measures of risk factors included task and postural analysis and electromyographic (EMG) evaluation of upper and lower trapezius muscles on some jobs. Workstation interventions initiated in 1975

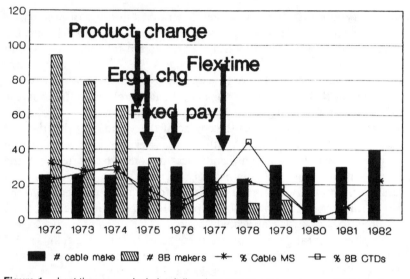

Figure 1. Lost time musculoskeletal disorders among cablemakers and 8B telephone cablemakers, 1972–1982, adapted from Westgaard and Aaras.[13,14]

included more adjustable height and slope of the work surfaces resulting in adopting suitable postures, arm rests on chairs and sit-stand alternatives. For example, in the 8B operation, percentage of EMG activity in the trapezius muscle at maximum voluntary contraction was reduced from 25% on the old system to 13% in the new workstation. The authors note a decline in both turnover and absences due to musculoskeletal problems after these interventions (Figure 1 adapted from Westgaard and Aaras).[13,14] While the authors believe the ergonomic changes were partially responsible for these "effects" among cablemakers and the 8B workers, they note a number of external and organizational changes that may have had a greater impact:

1. There was a product change which resulted in the gradual elimination of 8B jobs from approximately 90 in 1972 to 0 by 1981. This process began in 1975 (around the same time as the workstation changes). The evidence is a little more convincing for cablemakers where the number of jobs remained relatively constant over the study period. However, even in this job, a decrease in prevalence appears to have begun prior to workstation changes (Figure 1).

2. In 1976, shortly after the ergonomic interventions, a change in compensation took place in which fixed pay replaced an incentive sys-

tem. This may have resulted in less intensity of work and reduced psychosocial pressure.

3. Another major organizational change occurred in 1977 when flexible work times were introduced into the plant.

To try to estimate the impact of these various changes on outcome measures of musculoskeletal problems, absenteeism, and turnover, the investigators used questionnaire interviews with 100 employees. Of these:

- 55% reported a decrease in pain intensity.
- 41% thought their pain decrease was due to ergonomic adaptations.
- 45% had no decrease in pain but thought the workplace was better.
- 93% thought the best ergonomic change was the adjustable slope and height of the workbench.
- 73% thought the change to fixed pay was an important factor.
- 57% thought the improved work environment was responsible for the decreased turnover.

It is virtually impossible to sort out the contributions of any of the direct and indirect changes on reduction in musculoskeletal sick leaves in this study.

SOCIAL ISSUES

The Westgaard and Aaras investigation raises important work organization issues that many in-plant programs have ignored when trying to evaluate the impact of specific "small ergonomic interventions" on health outcomes.

1. In continuous flow processes where there is high process variability requiring rapid corrective action by employees, FLEXIBLE WORK GROUPS may be implemented, irrespective of any CTD control considerations.[7] This in turn may increase productivity through job elimination and decrease CTD risk factor exposure by essentially rotating workers through various tasks.

2. In traditional assembly and manufacturing operations, long flowlines may be shortened or abolished to increase flexibility in handling different products (irrespective of CTD control considerations). Productivity may be increased by a reduction in wait and material handling time. Quality may be improved by having the employees check their own work, thereby receiving more direct feedback.[7,15] The CTD risk factor of repetitiveness may be decreased by

having employees perform different tasks and motions; or it may be increased by eliminating rest (wait) times.

3. VERTICAL ROLE INTEGRATION combines roles such as set-up, production, and simple maintenance. It is used most often in white collar situations to improve productivity by improving morale, absenteeism, and turnover. Quality may improve due to more precise feedback and "intrinsic motivation." For example, repetitiveness may be decreased by having keypunch operators assume the added responsibility of supervising their own relationships with different departments whose work they process.

These organizational changes may meet the stated objectives of many in-plant ergonomic programs, but they are not without social costs. As Kelly[7] points out, there is often a substantial loss in jobs as a result. Employee acceptance of ergonomic changes is critical for effective interventions and perceived program success. If the cost of these changes is too great for employees (loss of jobs), participation in and acceptance of ergonomic programs will not be forthcoming, dooming most of them to failure.

SUMMARY

Ergonomic interventions to control CTDs do not occur in a vacuum. Changes in risk factors and reporting of CTDs may be affected as much by external factors (independent of specific ergonomic interventions) as any specific job changes. The types of interventions possible depend on existing technology, resources, and employee acceptance. Evaluation strategies must take into account limitations in exposure and outcome measures as well as recognize small numbers problems in statistical analyses. Although there are some promising evaluation measures such as postural discomfort type surveys that provide rapid feedback, their use as an early warning system for CTDs is still under investigation. Focusing on common risk factors rather than specific jobs may alleviate some of the sample size problems. When all is said and done, perceived success by management and employees may be the ultimate evaluation.

REFERENCES

1. Seashore, S.E., E.E. Lawler III, P.H. Mirvis and C. Cammann: *Assessing Organizational Change, A Guide to Methods, Measures & Practices.* John Wiley & Sons, New York (1984).

2. Fleiss, J.: *Statistical Methods for Rates and Proportions*, 2d ed. John Wiley & Sons, New York (1981).

3. Schlesselman, J.: *Case-Control Studies*. Oxford University Press, New York (1982).

4. Fine, L.J., B.A. Silverstein, T.J. Armstrong et al: Detection of Cumulative Trauma Disorders of Upper Extremities in the Workplace. *J. Occup. Med. 28(8)*:674–678 (1986).

5. Silverstein, B.A.: The Prevalence of Upper Extremity Cumulative Trauma Disorders in Industry. Ph.D. thesis. Epidemiologic Science, The University of Michigan, Ann Arbor (1985).

6. Sell, R.G.: Success and Failure in Implementing Changes in Job Design. *Ergonomics 23(8)*:809–816 (1980).

7. Kelly, J.E.: *Scientific Management, Job Redesign and Work Performance*. Academic Press, London (1982).

8. Stetson, D.S., T.J. Armstrong, L.J. Fine et al: A Survey of Chronic Upper Extremity Disorders in an Automobile Upholstery Plant. *Trends in Ergonomics/Human Factors III*, pp. 623–630. W. Karowski, Ed. Elsevier Science Publ., North Holland; New York (1986).

9. Corlett, E.N. and R.P. Bishop: A Technique for Assessing Postural Discomfort. *Ergonomics 19(2)*:175–182 (1976).

10. Karlqvist, L.: Cutting Operation at Canning Bench – A Case Study of Hand Tool Design. *Proceedings 1984 Intl. Conference on Occupational Ergonomics*, pp. 452–456. Toronto (1984).

11. Tannen, K.J., D.S. Stetson, B.A. Silverstein et al: An Evaluation of Scissors for Control of Upper Extremity Disorders in an Automobile Upholstery Plant. *Trends in Ergonomics/Human Factors III*, pp. 631–639. Op cit.

12. Webb, R.D.G. et al: Assessment of Musculoskeletal Discomfort in a Large Clerical Office – A Case Study. *Proceedings 1984 Intl. Conference on Occupational Ergonomics*, pp. 92–396, Toronto (1984).

13. Westgaard, R.H. and A. Aaras: Postural Muscle Strain as a Causal Factor in the Development of Musculo-skeletal Illnesses. *Appl. Ergonomics 15(3)*:162–174 (1984).

14. Westgaard, R.H. and A. Aaras: The Effect of Improved Workplace Design on the Development of Work-related Musculo-skeletal Illnesses. *Appl. Ergonomics 16*:91–97 (1985).

15. Hackman, J.R. and G.R. Oldham: *Work Redesign*. Addison Wesley, Reading, Massachusetts (1980).

CHAPTER 8

Detection of Cumulative Trauma Disorders of Upper Extremities in the Workplace

LAWRENCE J. FINE, M.D.,[A] **BARBARA A. SILVERSTEIN, Ph.D.,**[A]
THOMAS J. ARMSTRONG, Ph.D.,[A] **CHARLES A. ANDERSON, Ph.D.,**[B]
and DAVID S. SUGANO, Dr.P.H.[C]

[A]Department of Environmental and Industrial Health and Center for
Ergonomics, University of Michigan, Ann Arbor, Michigan; [B]Back System
Corporation, Dallas, Texas; [C]Health Systems and Surveillance Section,
Ford Motor Company, Dearborn, Michigan

This chapter addresses three issues: 1) the objectives and specific features of surveillance of upper extremities cumulative trauma disorders
(UECTDs) in the workplace, 2) the use of preexisting data sources
(PDSs) for surveillance of UECTDs, and 3) the use of questionnaire and
physical examination (QPE) data for surveillance. The principal objective of surveillance of UECTDs is to identify jobs with elevated rates of
disorders. In the past, this type of surveillance for UECTDs has largely
been restricted to research studies in contrast to other occupational
health problems such as noise-induced hearing loss, or occupational lung
diseases, for which surveillance activities have been routinely incorporated into occupational health programs.

Unlike some other occupational health disorders, UECTDs cannot
usually be detected in the presymptomatic state. Thus, although one

Published in *Journal of Occupational Medicine*, Vol. 28, No. 8, pp. 674–678, August 1986.
Copyright © by the American Occupational Medical Association. Reprinted with permis-
sion.

cannot screen for UECTDs, one can conduct surveillance programs for UECTDs. Surveillance for UECTDs is often easier than surveillance for other occupational disorders such as lung disease for three reasons. First, UECTDs are frequently more common than occupational lung disorders or occupational cancers. Second, in contrast to occupational lung diseases or cancers, UECTDs do not often have a substantial latency period. Third, workers will frequently work for considerable time periods with an active UECTD and as a result can be identified while they are still actively employed.

Within a plant, the relative risk of the "high-risk" jobs, regardless of data source, is frequently threefold to fivefold higher than the plant or baseline risk. The frequency of UECTDs make their surveillance feasible. A prevalence of 25/100 workers has been observed in our studies in a variety of industries such as the manufacturing of aircraft components using either QPE or with preexisting data sources.[1,2]

POSSIBLE OBJECTIVES OF SURVEILLANCE

The objectives of surveillance may be quite varied. Many investigators have used surveillance data to identify the causal determinants of UECTDs in the workplace. However, surveillance is more commonly used to identify the jobs with high rates of disorders so that an effective control program can be developed. Another use of a surveillance system is to determine if a control program is effective in achieving its objectives of reducing the number, severity, or cost of UECTDs. Costs of UECTDs are often calculated only on the basis of lost time or workers' compensation costs rather than using broader measures that assess the costs to the individual injured worker and costs due to lower levels of productivity. In our experience very few organizations can fully determine the costs of UECTDs. As a result, benefits of control activity are probably routinely underestimated.

In addition to analyzing causal associations, we have had the opportunity to address two other questions: 1) Can PDSs be used to identify jobs in plants with elevated rates of UECTDs? and 2) What is the sensitivity and specificity of a QPE surveillance program compared with the use of high-quality plant medical records?

METHODS

We have made frequent use of PDSs to identify the high-risk jobs within a plant. The preexisting data sources from one of our studies will be used to illustrate the answer to our first question. We analyzed the PDSs data from three large automobile manufacturing plants in the midwestern part of the United States (plants A, B, and C). We used one of four sources of data: 1) Occupational Safety and Health Administration (OSHA) 200 Logs; 2) workers' compensation records; 3) records of medical absences usually longer than 3 days or a week; 4) review of the plant medical records from plants A and B (medical cases). These data were collected over a 2- to 4-year period by the company. This particular firm had a central registry of all awarded worker compensation claims. All medical leaves resulting in an absence of 3 days or longer were also compiled in a central registry. The company coded the nature of these leaves according to the International Classification of Diseases Ninth classification scheme. In addition, we reviewed the medical records kept by the plant medical personnel which included a brief description of all disorders or injuries that might be work-related. Location and nature of the disorder (e.g., ganglion, carpal tunnel syndrome) as well as treatment were abstracted.

A computerized lifetime employment history initiated by the central occupational health personnel of this firm facilitated analysis. Once a month the current job of each employee was noted and his or her occupational history updated. By combining this exposure data with the above incidence data, job-specific incident rates were calculated. Job-specific rates were compared with the incident rate of all the other jobs at the specific plant by calculating the incidence density ratio (IDR), a measure of relative risk.

In order to answer the second question, we determined the sensitivity of QPE in detecting UECTDs diagnosed in the existing occupational medical records kept by a fourth plant from a different firm. Our QPE surveillance procedure consisted of three parts: 1) primary questionnaire, 2) supplemental symptomatic questionnaires, and 3) physical examination.

Primary Questionnaire

This questionnaire obtains information on demographic information, possible confounders, and effect modifiers. It is used to decide if the subject might have a cumulative trauma disorder (CTD) and if so, where the problem is located so that a symptomatic questionnaire can be filled out for that region of the body (shoulder/neck, elbow/forearm, or wrist/hand). Potential confounders include such variables as prior injuries, relevant diseases, or hobbies.

Symptomatic Questionnaire

This questionnaire provides more detailed information to establish whether, for surveillance purposes, a CTD is present, and what its severity and past treatment are. The patient draws on a diagram to localize the symptoms. Our past questionnaire criteria for a CTD required that the symptoms be present for longer than a week or occur more than 20 times in the previous year and not be the result of an acute injury. In the future we will separate the duration of each episode from the number of episodes over a one-year period.

Physical Examination

In developing our examination, we incorporated the elements of physical examinations used by experienced clinicians.[3-9] We wanted the examination to have the following characteristics: 1) to be more sensitive than specific because the objective of surveillance activities is usually the identification of jobs with high rates of disorders; 2) to require limited formal clinical training; and 3) to be limited in the time required to perform the evaluation. The design process attempted to break the examination into discrete steps and to describe each step precisely so that it could be performed by a nonexperienced clinician.

For each joint, starting with the neck and proceeding to the finger, we first decided which disorders we wanted to be able to detect. We included common disorders that occur frequently in the population but may not be considered a CTD, such as cervical intervertebral disc disorders. Identifying the disorders of interest required a relatively limited number of physical maneuvers or tests. Some parts of the examination only need to be performed if an abnormality is detected in an earlier part of the examination or if certain symptoms are present. The examination consists primarily of inspection, palpation, and passive, active, and resisted motions.

Examples of this flow sheet approach are the following: if the active range of motions of the neck is normal, then it is unnecessary to perform the passive motions. It is only necessary to check the pinprick sensation of the dermatomes of the arm if radicular pain is present; if there is appropriate muscle weakness; or if there are abnormalities of the deep tendon reflexes. This surveillance examination can be done in 15 to 30 minutes unless the subject has numerous complaints. By combining the information from the questionnaire and the physical examination we have defined diagnostic criteria. The criteria for de Quervain's disease are the following:

Interview: pain in anatomical snuffbox, may radiate up forearm. No history of fracture or radial wrist fracture. Lasting more than one week or more than 20 times in last year.

Physical Examination: rule out radial nerve entrapment, positive Finkelstein test with pain score of 4 or greater.

We have also used diagnostic criteria which are based solely on the questionnaire information. In this study we used the questionnaire definitions because we were interested in both active cases and resolved cases of CTDs. Usually we use the questionnaire and physical examination diagnostic criteria because we are primarily interested in identifying active cases.

Using our surveillance examination we surveyed 159 subjects in June 1983 who had been working for more than 1 year on one of eight jobs in an investment casting plant. The eight jobs were selected without knowledge of the health status of the workers from these jobs. The selection of jobs was based on the repetitiveness and forcefulness of the specific job tasks.[10] Ninety-five percent of the eligible workers participated in the survey. We then abstracted all the relevant information on the 159 workers from plant medical records. We believed that the current quality of these medical records with regard to CTDs was excellent whereas prior to middle 1981, they contained only limited information on CTDs. Between 1981 and early 1982, the medical records markedly improved, following a policy decision to establish a better surveillance system for CTDs. New nurses were hired and two physicians were contracted to provide part-time services. Cases of potential CTDs were often referred to a hand surgeon. Nurses were encouraged to record their findings regarding both acute trauma and CTDs. Out of the more than 20 different plant records we have collectively reviewed in the last 2 years, these records were among the best. Both sources (the medical records and the QPE survey) were independently evaluated for evidence of all types of recurring or persistent pain in the upper extremity, CTDs, and related disorders such as localized osteoarthrosis. The plant medical records were designated as the true indicator, whereas the surveillance examination was the test indicator.

TABLE I. High-Risk Jobs as Identified by Incidence Density Ratio (IDR) for Plant C
for All Types of Musculoskeletal Disorders and Injuries

Job Description	IDR*	P**
C Machine repair	28.2	.04
Repair rear seat back	24.4	.04
Seat back installation	11.9	.01
Grind and disk hammer-utility	9.6	.02
Motor decker	5.8	.05
Heater installation-utility	3.8	.05
Location-wide	1.0	

*Incidence density ratio (relative risk) = (no. of cases Job 1/h Job 1)/(All cases – Job
1)/(Total h – Job 1)
**x^2 df 1-, 2-tailed

TABLE II. Incident* by Plant by Source

	Plant	
Type of Disorder	B	C
Acute trauma		
OSHA	1.63	2.82**
Workers' Compensation	.33	.64
Medical Absence	1.96	2.00
Medical Cases	6.50	14.62**
Cumulative trauma disorders		
OSHA	.03	.15†
Workers' Compensation	.29	.45
Medical Absence	3.04	1.85**
Medical Cases	2.03	13.98**

*Incident rate = incidents per 100 worker-years.
**p < .005
†p < .05 (x^2 df 1-, 2-tailed)

RESULTS

Using either the medical absence or the medical case data, we were able
to identify jobs that had statistically significant elevated incidence density ratio (IDRs) (Table I). Our analysis of the PDSs illustrates some of
the limitations of these types of data. Most notable is the striking difference in the plantwide incident rates depending on which source one
examines (Table II). Some of this difference obviously occurs because
the sources differ on how severe the disorder must be in order for it to be
counted and whether the causal role of work is considered before it is
counted.

TABLE III.   Agreement of Records Regarding Upper Extremity Cumulative Trauma
Disorders*

Study Records	Disease	No Disease
Disease	59	50
No Disease	4	46
Total	63	96

*Sensitivity = 93.7%
Specificity = 47.9%
Positive predictive validity = 54.1%

The incidence rates between the two plants are different. Although this may in part be due to the nature of the specific jobs in each of the plants, it is more likely to be due to differences in the reporting policy of the two medical departments or other variables which do not reflect underlying rate of UECTD. Both plants assemble transportation equipment and are in the same state. This variability is likely to be even greater if one studies plants in different states because both local management policy and state laws will have a major impact on the relationship of the data sources to the underlying real rate of the problem. The incident rates from two of the sources (workers' compensation and OSHA) are quite low. This limits the usefulness of these sources for surveillance because only very high relative risks could be statistically detected unless several hundred worker-years of exposure per job can be analyzed.

As a result of our concerns about the limitations of using PDSs in surveillance and our research needs to be able to reliably determine the prevalence of UECTD in a variety of industries throughout the United States, we have been using a surveillance questionnaire and physical examination to estimate the prevalence of UECTD. Our experience with this approach suggests to us that it could be adapted for routine surveillance and would be superior to the use of PDSs. This led us to determine the sensitivity of our QPE when compared to existing occupational medicine records. As described earlier, we compared the results in QPE to the diagnoses in the medical records of 159 subjects from one plant.

Of the 159 subjects, 40 had no complaints related to the upper extremity (excluding abrasions and other acute trauma) in either of the indicators. The sensitivity was 93.7%, whereas the specificity was 47.9%, and the positive predicted validity was 54.1% (Table III). The large number of "false positives" is not surprising because we used the most sensitive definition of CTDs in this analysis (Table IV). We defined CTDs in terms of questionnaire-based diagnostic criteria. Thus, some of the conditions we found on our examination were mild (11 had no positive physical

TABLE IV. Diagnosis of "False Positives"

Diagnosis	No. of Workers
Carpal tunnel syndrome	7
Nonspecific hand/wrist	5
Rheumatoid arthritis	6
Nonspecific elbow/forearm	6
Shoulder tendinitis	4
Nonspecific shoulder	6
Neck/scapular tension	18
Ganglions	2
Osteoarthrosis	2
Thoracic outlet syndrome	2

findings) and may not have been severe enough for the workers to seek medical assistance. Twenty-eight of these workers whose results were "false-positive" noted on their questionnaire that they had not sought any treatment for their conditions. In addition, seven had been treated by chiropractors. Some of the diagnoses rested on signs of localized osteoarthritis in the distal joints of the fingers. These diagnoses were not noted in the plant records. For the other diagnosis, neck/scapular tension, for which there were a large number of "false positives," there are few widely accepted diagnostic criteria. We defined this condition as diffuse or localized pain in the muscles of the dorsal aspect of the neck or the upper part of the trapezius muscle, usually associated with localized areas of muscle tenderness or spasm and increased pain on resisted lateral flexion or rotation of the neck.[11-13] If we exclude all of the "false-positive" workers who never sought treatment from any health care provider, then our "adjusted" specificity improves to 73% and our positive predictive validity to 81% (Table V).

The results of the comparison of the surveillance examination with the plant medical records revealed a high level of agreement for most CTDs. Only over the diagnoses of localized osteoarthrosis in the joints of the fingers and tension neck syndrome was there substantial disagreement.

In summary, each of the two approaches of surveillance of UECTD has its advantages and disadvantages (Table VI). It is too early in our comparison of PDSs systems with QPE to reach final conclusions. It is clear that a QPE system can be as sensitive as an excellent plant medical department in detecting UECTD. Many plant medical records are not kept in sufficient detail or with sufficient consistency in recording of diagnoses to permit detailed surveillance for UECTD. Nevertheless, the low cost of a PDSs system is an attraction.

Also with a preexisting data sources system, retrospective analyses can

TABLE V.   Adjusted Results of the Screening Examination*

| Study Records | Plant Records | |
	Disease	No Disease
Disease	59	15
No Disease	4	46
Total	63	61

*"Adjusted" Sensitivity = 93.7%
  "Adjusted" Specificity = 73%
  "Adjusted" Positive predictive validity = 81%
  Table excludes workers who never sought medical treatment.

TABLE VI.   Comparison of Preexisting Data Sources (PDSs) with Questionnaire and Physical Examination (QPE) for Surveillance

PDS	QPE
Advantages	
Low cost	Better for multiple sites
May allow retrospective analyses	Collects information on confounders and effect modifiers
	May be less biased
	May be more sensitive
Disadvantages	
Often insensitive, biased, or nonexistent	Requires training of medical personnel
Requires review of medical records	More costly than PDSs

potentially be more readily conducted. QPE requires that workers be examined periodically and that standard methods of examination be used. An organization that used QPE would need some experience with its interpretation. QPE can be used to obtain information on potential confounders and effect modifiers. Greater experience with both PDSs and QPE systems for surveillance will need to be obtained before it will be clear which one is superior for a particular surveillance need. It is likely that a combination approach will prove to be the most effective surveillance strategy.

REFERENCES

1. McGlothlin, J.D., T.F. Armstong, L.J. Fine et al: Can Job Changes Initiated by a Joint Labor-Management Task Force Reduce the Prevalence and Incidence of Cumulative Trauma Disorders of the Upper Extremity? *Proceedings of the 1984 International Conference on Occupational Ergonomics*, Vol. 1, pp. 336–340. Human Factor Conference Inc., Rexdale, Canada (1984).
2. Silverstein, B.A., L.J. Fine, T.J. Armstrong and B. Joseph: The Effects of Forceful and Repetitive Work on the Upper Extremity. *Proceedings of the 1984 International Conference on Occupational Ergonomics*, Vol. 1, pp. 351–355. Human Factor Conference Inc., Rexdale, Canada (1984).
3. Brown, P.: Peripheral Nerve Lesions. *Musculoskeletal Disorders: Regional Examination and Differential Diagnosis*, p. 147. D'Ambrosia, Ed. J.B. Lippincott, Philadelphia (1977).
4. Cailliet, R.: *Soft Tissue Pain and Disability*. F.A. Davis Co., Philadelphia (1980).
5. Cailliet, R.: *Hand Pain and Impairment*. F.A. Davis Co., Philadelphia (1975).
6. Cailliet, R.: *Neck and Arm Pain*. F.A. Davis Co., Philadelphia (1981).
7. Cailliet, R.: *Neck and Arm Pain*, 2d ed. F.A. Davis Co., Philadelphia (1981).
8. Cailliet, R.: *Shoulder Pain*. F.A. Davis Co., Philadelphia (1981).
9. Cyriax, J.: *Textbook of Orthopaedics*, 7th ed. Baillier Tindall, London (1979).
10. Silverstein, B.A., L.J. Fine and T.J. Armstrong: Hand-wrist Cumulative Trauma Disorders in Industry. *Brit. J. Ind. Med.* (in press 1986).
11. Waris, P.: Occupational Cervicobrachial Syndromes: A review. *Scand. J. Work Environ. Health 6(suppl.)*:3–14 (1980).
12. Maeda, K.: Occupational Cervicobrachial Disorders in Assembly Plants. *Kuruma Med. J. 22*:231 (1975).
13. Valtonen E: The Tension Neck Syndrome: Its Etiology, Clinical Features and Results of Physical Treatment. *Ann. Med. Mil. Fenn. 57*:139–142 (1968).

CHAPTER 9

Design of Hand Tools for Control of Cumulative Trauma Disorders

STEPHEN W. MEAGHER, M.D.

520 Commonwealth Avenue, Boston, Massachusetts 02215

Before iron was made available to native Americans, they had to fashion all of their tools from stone, bone, wood, and shell. They had to consider hardness, size, shape, length, purpose, frictional characteristics, weight, and comfort in fashioning necessary tools. These elements have endured as the primary human factor elements of tool design today.

Many examples exist that demonstrate the intelligent craftsmanship that preceded the appearance of the white man in North America. Striking, prying, twisting, weaving, scraping, cutting, drawing, and agricultural tools were produced in various configurations.

The freedom of modern designers to do as they please according to their individual abilities has resulted in design errors that cause cumulative trauma disorders (CTDs) through misuse of basic tool design elements. It is essential for designers to understand the features of human anatomy that make the hand vulnerable to inappropriate use of tool design elements.

The application of skin to a tool handle can result in CTDs because of the elements of thickness, dryness, excessive moisture, smoothness, and individual response to abrasive surfaces.[1,2] The adverse effect of excessive pressure upon underlying structures is enhanced by thin skin with resultant muscle soreness and eventual muscle spasm.

Dry and very wet skin result in difficult tool retention with a dissipation of energy that would have been transmitted into the task otherwise. When there is a weak bonding between the hand and handle, intrinsic muscle strains can result and produce temporary disability.

Thin skin and to a lesser extent thick skin cannot withstand a repetitive abrasive force without pain or actual abrasion such as is encountered with a chipped tool handle or a plastic handle with a mold seam that has not been polished off. A strong tool maintenance program is always necessary.

Broad, deep fluting of handles grabs areas of skin and fascia, traumatizing them during forceful rotary movement[3] as encountered in the use of screwdrivers and manual nut drivers. The resulting discomfort diminishes efficiency and prevents maximum input of energy into the task.

The absence of significant padding by fat at skin creases over the middle and end joints of the fingers exposes the underlying tendons, tendon sheaths, and joint capsules to injury from angular tool handles and bare metal bar stock or narrow handles which are held with the fingers moderately extended. In very small diameter handles, the fat pads of the fingers come together and protect skin crease areas from harm.

The length and breadth of the female hand are not greatly different from the male hand. However, the circumference of the female hand is of greater importance anthropometrically because it reflects the smaller muscle mass and bone structure of the female hand. Light muscling of the hand exposes underlying structures to percussion and compression injuries. Because strength is related directly to muscle mass[4] one can readily understand why the lightly muscled female hand has difficulty with heavy tools.

The increasing participation of women in utility line work, general construction and unskilled general labor brings them into a confrontation with loppers, sledge hammers, chippers, picks, shovels, heavy wire cutters, and other tools which have been designed for use by the stronger male hand in the past. The large diameter handles on some of these tools and the forceful use of large loppers around utility poles with arms abducted and elbows flexed result in assorted intrinsic muscle strains, myositis, straining of hand and wrist ligaments, and epicondylitis.

The bulk of the workforce in electronic assembly operations is made up of female employees who have considerable difficulty with pliers, wire strippers, and pistol grip tools when they are used extensively. Triggers on pistol grip tools that exercise only the index finger are more apt to cause trigger fingers and muscle strain due to locking of the other digits on the handle for prolonged periods. Handle length triggers that permit exercising of all four fingers intermittently during the use of the tool can alleviate this problem.

It is desirable to distribute handle pressure over a large area of skin contact to prevent a concentration of force against a small area of skin with severe compression of underlying structures.

The weaker female hand can be partially addressed by using tool length, precision machining, lubrication, Teflon-like coatings on moving surfaces of hand tools and an excellent tool maintenance program.

Tool handles should conform to hand contours, present a broad surface to the hand and be long enough to span the poorly padded central palm to avoid compression injuries of intrinsic muscles and neurovascular elements.

Hand tools can cause serious injury to nerves and arteries through exposure to vibration from tools such as grinders, sanders, chippers, power saws, and other tools. Vibration is a problem in machine processing of hand-held stock. The condition of "white finger" is caused by vibration and is manifested by blanching of skin, coldness, numbness, and pain. Prolonged exposure to vibration can cause irreversible changes in vascular and neural elements. The appearance of "white finger" is an indication for withdrawal from use of the tool.

The use of striking tools can cause clotting within an artery of the hand and produce a "hammer syndrome"[5] which produces sensitivity to cold, impaired strength of grasp, and easy fatigability of the hand. Because of this problem, shock absorbance of the handles of striking tools is essential. At zero shock absorbance, the force of each blow is transmitted into the hand as well as into the task.

Direct contusion of the median and ulnar nerve branches in the palm can be caused by pounding with the palm on a stiff tool such as an addressograph printer for credit cards. Fine tools that require the thumb ray to be flexed across the palm can produce a carpal tunnel syndrome. Cases which are thought to be carpal tunnel syndrome from hand tools are far more often due to contusion or compression injuries of median nerve branches in the proximal palm given off as the median nerve emerges from the carpal tunnel. In an industrial setting, carpal tunnel syndromes are usually due to abnormal work performance movements, not to the tool that is being used.

The skeletal elements of the hand are tightly tethered to one another by ligaments that ensure joint stability and efficient movement during the function of tendon-muscle units. All ligaments of the hand and upper extremity are vulnerable to injury from the chronic stresses applied to them by unsupported heavy tools, torquing action of power tools, and forceful rotary use of hand tools such as wrenches and rotary jack handles. Localized tenderness over the ligament and pain when tensing the involved ligament by passive or active movements is present. The most commonly injured ligament is the medial collateral ligament at the base of the thumb which is chronically stressed by a large tool handle and plier type handles.

Joint capsules with their inner secretory synovial lining can be injured by ring handles and forceful use of a wide variety of hand tools. Arthritic joints in the fingers and wrist are especially vulnerable to aggravation with resulting swelling, tenderness, restricted range of motion, and pain when severe.[3]

It is very important to remember that the tissues of each individual have a threshold of resistance to pathological change. If that threshold is crossed by too many units of work with a defective tool in a unit of time over a period of time pathological changes will appear.[6] This principle

TABLE I.   Examples of Cumulative Trauma Disorders Caused by Hand Tools

Sex	Tool	C.T.D.
M	Hand sander	Trigger fingers (2); tingling I M R S; tender palm
F	Crimping tool	Synovitis radial wrist
	Cutting tool	Myositis ext. muscles
F	Labelmatic gun	Bilateral carpal tunnel syndrome (CTS) (pricing groceries)
F	Addressograph printer	Stiffness (pounding keys); contusion; chronic pain thumb ray
F	Ticket gun (labeling shoes)	Trigger thumb; aggravation of arthritis
F	Crimping tool, strong opening spring	Strain MP joint thumb
M	Hard flex rubber to put sealant into joints of auto	Swollen index; strained joints (index finger)
M	Whiz knife (12 hams/10 sec)	Trigger fingers (2)
F	Hammer (framing)	Epicondylitis
F	Ships (cutting wood strips)	Tenosynovitis; intrinsic muscle strain; swelling
F	Welding gun, strong spring loaded cord (use under rear deck of auto)	Myositis, peripheral nerve stretch injury
F	Tweezers and pliers (repairing sockets)	Neuritis, burning pain in hand
M	Floor polisher	Neuritis, dullness to midforearms, vasospasm, roniacol relieved
F	Pneumatic dental polisher; hand scaling	Bilateral CTS, (ganglia over flex, rad. longus insertion)

provides a logical basis for work rotation schedules which provide a variety of physical movements.

Hand tools can cause the following cumulative disorders: trigger finger, capsulitis, neuritis, myositis, synovitis, stenosing tenovaginitis, tendinitis, ligament strain or attenuation, muscle strain, carpal tunnel syndrome, brachial plexus stretch injury, thoracic outlet syndrome, arterial injury, periostitis, muscle strain, joint subluxation, epicondylitis, and aggravation of arthritis. Some of these disorders result from using heavy tools with the arms in an elevated position for prolonged periods of time. Examples of reported CTDs caused by specific hand tools are listed in Table I.

SUMMARY

A variety of cumulative trauma disorders can be caused by hand tools. Even when tool design elements are correct, a tool can still produce a disorder by being used too frequently in a unit of time over a period of time. The possibility of causing a cumulative trauma disorder is enhanced by errors in design related to tool handle size, shape, length, texture, shock absorbance, ease of use, and weight.

REFERENCES

1. Armstrong, T.: Mechanical Considerations of Skin in Work. *Am. J. Ind. Med.* 8:463–472 (1985).
2. Naylor, P.: The Skin Surface and Reaction. *Brit. J. Derm.* 67:239–248 (1955).
3. Meagher, S.: Hand Tools: Cumulative Trauma Disorders Caused by Improper Use of Design Elements. *Trends in Ergonomics/Human Factors III*, pp. 581–587. W. Karwowski, Ed. Elsevier, North Holland; New York (1986).
4. Sullivan, J. et al: The Properties of Skeletal Muscle. *Ortho. Review XV*, 6:349/17–363/31 (1986).
5. Benedict, K. et al: The Hypothenar Hammer Syndrome. *Radiol.* 111:57–60 (1974).
6. Meagher, S.: Wear and Tear: A Popular Fallacy. *Boston Bar. J. Oct.*, pp. 7–11 (1971).

CHAPTER 10

Ergonomic Considerations: Engineering Controls at Volkswagen of America

MAQUIS ECHARD, STEVE SMOLENSKI and **MICHAEL ZAMISKA**

Volkswagen of America, Inc., Westmoreland Assembly Plant, New Stanton, Pennsylvania

HISTORY OF ERGONOMIC DEVELOPMENT AT VOLKSWAGEN WESTMORELAND AND PRESENT TASK FORCE MAKEUP

During the latter part of 1981, injuries such as carpal tunnel syndrome (CTS), tendonitis, and lower back strain began to show a significant increase according to the accident and injury reports at the Westmoreland facility (Figure 1). One area of particular concern was the seat and cushion build area of the Chassis Department. A statistical analysis of the seat area found that CTS had escalated to almost epidemic proportions accounting for 62% of the Chassis Department's total experience. As a result of these findings, a special task force of local United Auto Workers and management members was authorized and assigned the task of investigating CTS in the seat and cushion build area. The group, known as the "Carpal Tunnel Committee," was successful in reducing CTS in the seat build area to 14% of the Chassis Department's experience of 10 to 14 cases per year (Figure 2). However, the committee, as originally designed, developed various inefficiencies due to the large size (10 members), limited training, and lack of broad base support by management members. These problems slowed the expansion of the committee into other areas of cumulative trauma disorders and the broadening of committee involvement on a plantwide basis. These inadequacies were overcome through a streamlining of the committee to enhance communi-

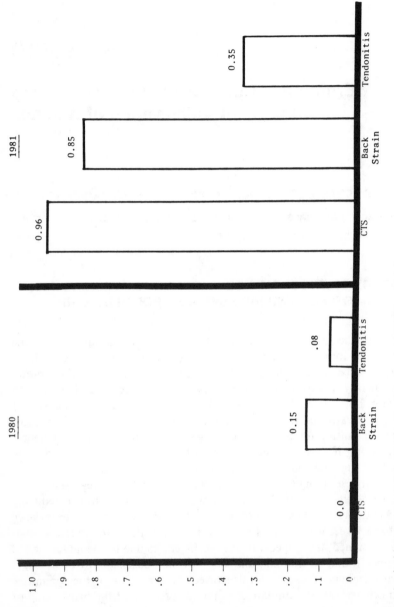

Figure 1. Incident rates per 100 employees using standard OSHA calculations.

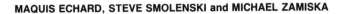

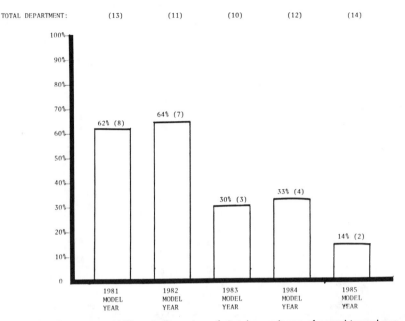

Figure 2. Percentage of Chassis Department's total experience of carpal tunnel syndrome found in the seat/cushion room.

cations and responsibility and to build the educational and training base of both committee members and plant personnel.

The Joint VW/UAW Ergonomics Task Force, as it is known today, consists of five members representing Medical, Engineering, Safety, and Benefits, with full support, both financial and moral, from members of management and union to achieve the desired quality of their product and health of their people (Figure 3).

JOB EVALUATION—METHODS AND APPLICATIONS

In evaluating and classifying tasks at Volkswagen Westmoreland, the traditional methods-time measurements (MTM) system is used. However, all Volkswagen Westmoreland Planners and Design personnel are given a basic overview of an ergonomic outlook and evaluation of job design. This in-house training is given so that the personnel responsible for the actual job and tool design can understand and apply ergonomic concepts and principles. The engineering intent of the training is to blend the traditional methods of task analysis with the evermore important

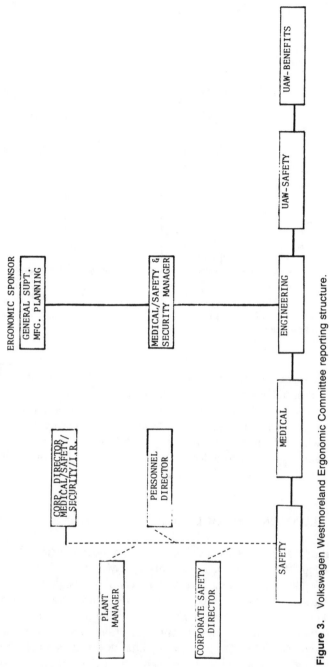

Figure 3.   Volkswagen Westmoreland Ergonomic Committee reporting structure.

outlook of the human factors. The training consists of human factors, job design, anthropometry, and strength/endurance. With this information and criteria, the engineers can evaluate the task first with a macro design outlook and apply creative solutions to reach the input and output catalysts needed to perform the desired task requirements.

SELECTED JOB ANALYSIS

Gas Filler Neck Boot Install

Work Description: Read manifest, install plug to filler neck boot, open filler neck door and remove cap, install fuel tank filler neck boot to filler neck by hand, install filler neck boot to inner fender panel with retainer ring, install gravity valve nipple to filler neck boot.

Summary of Problem: Case involves a male worker who collected compensation for approximately eight months due to a cervical strain allegedly received while working the gas filler neck boot operation. After several months on the operation, the employee reported to the Medical Department complaining of neck and shoulder pain and was diagnosed as having an acute cervical strain with shoulder tendonitis.

As shown in Figure 4a, the 31-year-old, 5'9" male worker's head is hyperextended, with both arms fully extended at a 170-degree angle in comparison to the worker's midline for approximately 50 seconds per unit; a 10-second fatigue recovery time is allotted between units.

Recommendations: Move operation from current location to the Final IV line where the work height would be 170 cm off the floor compared to the current 200 cm height (Figure 4b).

Underbody Wax Spray

Work Description: Close bumper reinforcement holes with covers, spray wax to front bumper reinforcement holes — nozzle #1, spray wax to front bumper reinforcement holes — nozzle #2, spray wax to front long member through wheelhouse liner hole — nozzle #3, spray wax to front long member lower section — nozzle #4, spray wax to rear long member — nozzle #14, remove bumper reinforcement hole covers.

Summary of Problem: Case involves several workers complaining of fatigue and discomfort of the upper extremities as a result of spraying wax in dead space areas under the units. An ergonomic review of the

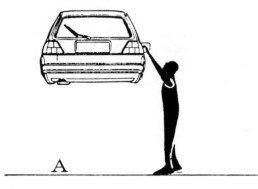

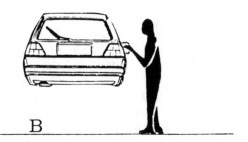

Figure 4. Gas filler neck boot installation; A, before and B, after implementation of recommendations.

operation (Figure 5a) shows the worker's shoulder angle at or around 80 to 90 degrees; the elbow angle is at 90 degrees while holding a 5-pound gun and hose for a 38- to 42-second period; recovery time between units is only eight to nine seconds.

Recommendations: The following two suggestions made by the task force were designed to eliminate the weight of the gun and hose from the operator's hand (Figure 5b).

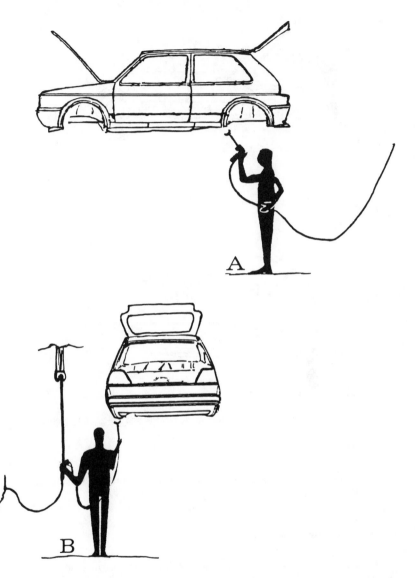

Figure 5. Underbody wax spray operation; A, before and B, after implementation of recommendations.

1. Attach the gun trigger mechanism and hose to a belt around the operator's waist with a single light wand to apply wax.
2. Suspend the gun trigger mechanism and hose from the overhead

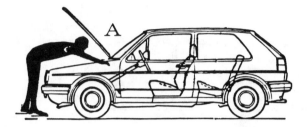

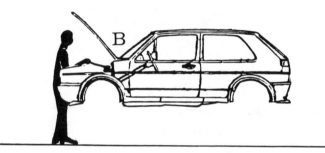

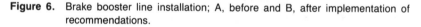

Figure 6. Brake booster line installation; A, before and B, after implementation of recommendations.

trolley system, eliminating the weight of the current gun and use a single, lightweight wand to apply wax.

Brake Booster Line Install

Work Description: The brake booster line install is only one element of the battery secure operation. Other elements involve securing positive and negative terminals and securing the battery cover.

Summary of Problem: Case involves a 33-year-old female worker diagnosed as having bilateral carpal tunnel syndrome after working the brake booster line install in our Final area for approximately one year. An ergonomic evaluation of this operation shows (Figure 6a) the 5′4″ female worker leaning over the front engine compartment with both arms/

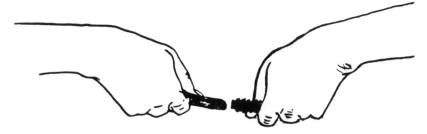

Figure 7.   Manual assembly of gas line hoses.

hands extended forward reaching for the brake booster line. Once in hand, the worker must push the hose end into the brake booster canister located on the driver side firewall at 56 cm off the floor. Because of the force needed to insert the hose end, the employee feels she must use the palms of her hands which results in hyperextension of the hand when securing the hose.

Recommendation: First design a tool to assist the worker in inserting the hose end. Secondly, although no complaints concerning back pain were received, the possibility for back trauma to develop from bending into the engine compartment was quite possible. Therefore, the operation should be moved to a location prior to bumper and radiator install, allowing the worker to walk within inches of the booster canister. The booster canister location is now 98 cm off the floor, requiring no excessive bending over the engine (Figure 6b).

Gas Line Subassembly

Work Description: Pick up sender hose in left hand and return pipe in right, secure sender hose to return pipe (twist on), secure hose to other end of return line with one clamp, pick up sender hose in left hand and feed pipe in left, secure the two (twist on), secure hose to other end of feed line with one clamp (Figure 7).

Summary of Problem: This 55-year-old female worker developed hand/wrist pain and numbness which was diagnosed as bilateral carpal tunnel syndrome. Reviewing the operation, the worker is seen using a pinch grip with excessive flexing of the wrists for a build of 1000 per day.

Recommendations: Design a tool where the hose and hose connectors can be secured with one smooth movement of a lever system.

Carburetor Adjustment, Engine Hot Test

Work Description: Operation consists of attaching two electrical probe clamps to engine, read digital display, determine adjustment need, adjust carburetor set screw (located on top of engine) while monitoring display.

Summary of Problem: In this case, the workers were complaining of pain and discomfort to their neck and shoulder areas after several hours on this operation. Upon reviewing the job site, we find the worker's arms fully extended at a 100-degree angle out over the top of the hot running engine while setting the carburetor adjustment screw. During this adjustment procedure, the operator's head is turned to the right at an angle between 70 and 120 degrees, depending on the position of the moving hot test line and the digital display box, which is located five feet to the operator's right side and at a height of seven feet from the floor (Figure 8a).

Recommendations: Move the digital display box inward, four feet closer to the worker and at a height where the operator's head will be in a forward, neutral position. The use of a long-handled flexible screwdriver was also suggested (Figure 8b).

Ashtray to Door Panel Install

Work Description: Get door pad from container, step to fixture, place pad in fixture, get tray from table, place tray in fixture, place screwdriver end over tray lugs, apply pressure to handle, withdraw screwdriver, apply screwdriver to second lug, apply pressure to handle, remove pad from fixture, step to cart, place pad in cart.

Summary of Problem: After performing the operation for several months, a 5' female worker developed pain to an area on the side of the wrist at the base of the thumb, which was diagnosed as de Quervain's disease. Reviewing the operation, we see severe ulnar wrist deviation while the worker presses the screwdriver against the lugs (Figure 9).

Recommendations: Design fixture that will press the ashtray into the door pad with one smooth movement of the upper extremity.

Vent Window Subassembly/Install

Work Description: Remove glass vent from box, place vent into fixture, remove rib from box, place rib on edge of glass, secure rib to glass using mallet, remove vent glass and rib from fixture, set in door window frame, secure using mallet.

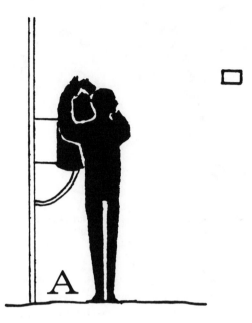

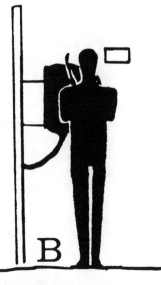

Figure 8. Carburetor adjustment, engine hot test; A, before and B, after implementation of recommendations.

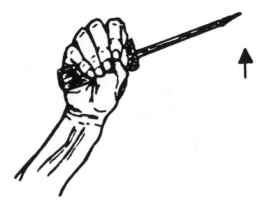

Figure 9.   Force and technique required to install ashtray to door panel before implementation of recommendations.

Summary of Problem: In this case, several Trim Department employees developed elbow and hand pain diagnosed as epicondylitis and carpal tunnel syndrome as a result of excessive swinging of the mallet (elbow movement) and grasping in combination with vibration of the mallet.

Recommendations: Press the rib and vent glass together using a pneumatic press.

Window Washer Line, Subassembly/Install

Work Description: Cut front washer tee to washer bottle hose to length, cut left-hand front washer tee to spray nozzle hose to length, cut right front washer tee to spray nozzle hose to length, subassemble sleeve to both ends of the left-hand washer nozzle spray hose, subassemble sleeve to both ends of the front washer tee to washer bottle hose, subassemble sleeve to both ends of the right washer nozzle spray hose, subassemble the three washer hoses (one grommet and one tee), install four clips to the hood for mounting the front washer nozzle and reservoir hoses, route the washer hose/tee subassembly through four clips, seat the grommet in the plenum and connect to nozzle, connect the front reservoir hose to the front reservoir, and finally hook up harness connector to front.

Summary of Problem: While performing the operation, all the workers in this area experienced upper extremity hand/wrist pain and discomfort diagnosed as digital neuritis along with carpal tunnel syndrome. Upon reviewing this operation, several unnatural hand/wrist postures

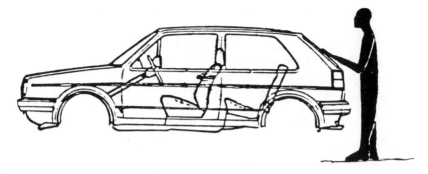

Figure 10. General posture needed to install rear hatch glass.

were noted including repetitious flexing and twisting of both wrists as well as cutting pressures to the digits. All resulted from use of spring-handled spreaders while performing the subassembly aspect of this operation.

Recommendations: Design system to spread and complete several hose systems (both ends) at one time, while eliminating unnatural hand/wrist postures and cutting effects of digits.

Rear Hatch Glass Install

Work Description: Employee applies slip agent to rubber seal around the edge of glass, grasps the glass on each side, lifts glass from stock and carries to vehicle; glass is then aligned with the opening and the rubber seal started in the metal channel; as one employee pulls the seating string from inside the vehicle, another employee pushes on glass and pounds glass to seat the rubber seal in position (Figure 10).

Summary of Problem: The employee uses a standard 3-inch paint brush to apply the slip agent on the dry rubber seal. This requires a pinching action to hold the brush with arm and shoulder extension to reach the back side of the glass, and wrist rotation to follow around the edge. The glass is then picked up by the edges using a pinch grip of the thumb and four fingers and placed in the hatch opening. Wrist extension is used to start the rubber seal in the metal channel with pressure applied using the palm of the hand. Pounding on the glass is done with open palms and requires considerable pressure to seat glass completely. String puller inside unit pulls on string to seat glass and wraps excess string around hand in time with pounding activity.

Recommendations: Temporary solutions may include the following:

1. Application of the slip agent does not require excessive stress except grasping of the brush. A heavy rubber glove is worn to prevent skin contact with the slip agent, which increases the force necessary to hold the brush which has a small handle. A swab-type brush should be used with a long handle that can be bent on an angle to decrease force needed to hold and reduce wrist deviation.

2. Grasping the glass to place into hatch is compounded due to slip agent reducing the gripping friction requiring additional force to hold and position glass. Suction cup grippers should be provided to prevent hand contact with slip agent and decrease hand strength needed to hold glass.

3. Pushing on the glass and hammering into place results in excessive shock to the palm area. Palm pads should be provided to reduce hand trauma.

Long-term planning should include:

1. Investigation into rubber seal around glass. Currently, seal is not preformed to glass and is dry requiring slip agent. Seal should be preformed and prelubricated to enhance fit and eliminate slip agent usage.

2. Develop fixture to seat glass, eliminating hand pounding currently performed.

3. Develop one-way, dog-type hand tool for the string pull operation. Current hand pulling and wrapping of string around hand should be eliminated.

SUMMARY

Thanks to an active ergonomic program of early detection education, improved medical treatment, and engineering controls, today at Volkswagen of America, we have been able to significantly reduce long-term disabilities associated with cumulative trauma disorders of the upper extremities and back, along with a 50% reduction in the need for surgical intervention of carpal tunnel syndrome in the early to moderate stages.

ACKNOWLEDGMENT

We would like to thank the management group at Volkswagen of America for their full support, both financial and moral, of the ergonomic endeavor by the task force. Also, we would like to thank the International UAW and Local 2055 officials and members for their continued support and activities as members of the Joint VW/UAW Ergonomics Task Force. A special thanks to Toolmaker, Frank Kinkela for his assistance in design, fabrication, and modification of fixtures and trick tools.

REFERENCES

Occupational Ergonomics, June 11–15, 1984, T.J. Armstrong and D.B. Chaffin Co-Chairmen. University of Michigan, College of Engineering, Engineering Summer Conferences. Information obtained from course material which included the following references: D.S. Bloswick, P.E., Ph.D. Candidate; G.D. Herrin, Ph.D.; T.G. Hiebert, M.D., Ph.D.; K.W. Kennedy, Ph.D.; G.G. Langolf, Ph.D.; R.G. Radwin, M.S., M.S.E. and C.B. Woolley, M.S.

CHAPTER 11

Analysis of a Program for Control of Cumulative Trauma Disorders in the Auto Industry

BRADLEY S. JOSEPH, Ph.D.

The Medical College of Ohio, Department of Occupational Health, School of Allied Health, C.S. 10008, Toledo, Ohio

INTRODUCTION

Despite years of ergonomic research, an abundance of technical information, and evidence that using ergonomics in job designs reduces the incidence of injury,[1,2] ergonomics, by and large, has not been adequately incorporated into the workplace. Consequently, many industries suffer from increased incidence of musculoskeletal disorders, decreased productivity, and worker dissatisfaction.

It is hypothesized that ergonomics has not been adequately incorporated into the workplace for a variety of reasons. Two important reasons are outlined in this chapter. First, ergonomics is a multidisciplinary science. One company defines their goals in ergonomics as "the integration and application of scientific disciplines, such as physiology, psychology, and engineering in designing and improving the workplace to minimize errors, reduce the risk of accidents or chronic injuries while increasing employee well-being, product quality, and productivity." Accomplishing this goal requires effective input from a variety of diverse specialties both inside and outside the organization.

Second, traditional organizations in many industries have erected barriers that reduce successful mixing of disciplines that are essential in designing and implementing sound ergonomics. These barriers include a lack of general ergonomic knowledge within those disciplines of the organization that must be included in ergonomic decisions, a lack of job knowledge about the job that should be changed, communication break-downs between disciplines, and subunit interest (organizational units that have their own self-interest in mind).[3]

One approach to overcoming these barriers is through the use of cross-functional ergonomic task forces designed to bring together representa-tives from the necessary disciplines needed for good ergonomic design. Research suggests that group decisionmaking processes are an effective way to manage technical change.[4,5] To determine the effectiveness of this approach, an ergonomic control program using a participative task force approach was implemented in a large American automotive parts plant.

There are several ways to evaluate the successfulness of such pro-grams; however, resource constraints usually limit the number of ways. Several criteria used to evaluate this program are discussed. First, the effectiveness of the training in teaching participants the basic principles of ergonomics and job design/redesign was monitored to determine if the groups have the necessary knowledge to make job changes. Second, participants' perceptions of meetings were investigated to study their satisfaction with the program. Third, the number and quality of job changes were monitored to determine the effectiveness of the groups in making job changes. Finally, the effectiveness of the program in reduc-ing the incidence of injury related to ergonomic stress is being analyzed.

This chapter concentrates on evaluating the program from the first and second perspective. Suffice it to say that the program resulted in many job changes over a one and one-half year time frame. Reductions in the incidence of injury occur only after the job redesigns have been implemented. Data is now being collected to study the effects of job change on the incidence of injury.

Why evaluate ergonomic training and participant perceptions of meet-ings in the context of a participative ergonomic program? There are several reasons. Ergonomic training is designed to give participants an in-house expertise of ergonomic principles used in job design. Several companies are now sending in-house staff to training seminars to gain the necessary knowledge and to develop and implement ergonomic changes in their workplaces. After the training, companies expect these persons to be able to set up, organize, run, and implement ergonomic programs in the workplace. However, often the most important knowl-edge base for these practitioners is a combination of the knowledge gained in these ergonomic courses and in the personal experience that comes from using the knowledge on the plant floor, raising obvious questions about the competence of these "practitioners" to effectively do the things the corporations expect of them after they complete these courses. In this regard, several questions concerning ergonomic knowledge learned during training courses is important to know in the development of effective training in the future. In particular:

1. What level of ergonomic knowledge already exists in the plant?

2. Was there a general increase in ergonomic knowledge after the training?

3. How did participants' level of education or years of industrial experience affect their existing ergonomic knowledge or the amount they learned from the training?

Why evaluate participant perceptions in the context of participative ergonomics programs? Participant perceptions are important measures of the success of the program for three reasons:

First, common sense reasoning would have one believe that ergonomic meetings, or any meetings, that participants view as a waste of time and not in their best interest for career development would not have the support of the participants. This lack of commitment would seriously hamper the effectiveness of the group in getting things done and the ultimate and long-term success of the program.[6]

Second, information about perceptions of participants intimately involved in a group in the program is very important in determining the effectiveness of the group. Participants who are not satisfied with the program and choose not to participate or choose to censor their ideas will adversely affect the overall effectiveness of the group because a prerequisite for effective group decisionmaking is the careful consideration of dissenting viewpoints.[7,8] Careful analysis of participant perceptions may uncover the reason for these problems.

Third, ergonomic programs involving group decisionmaking have dual objectives: satisfaction of the goals of the program and satisfaction of the participants who are involved in the program.[6] Programs that achieve the ergonomic objectives, at the expense of the participants by frustrating the people that make it work, are only partly successful. Likewise, programs that satisfy group members' needs, but do not accomplish anything substantial, are also not successful. Therefore, like quality of worklife programs, ergonomics programs involving participation need to be monitored through participants' perceptions to ensure that both objectives are being fulfilled.

In summary, participants' satisfaction with meetings can give information about what makes a successful meeting. Several issues that are important in dealing with this question are:

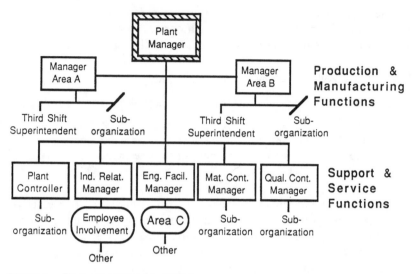

Figure 1. Plant operating organization.

1. Was attendance at meetings associated with participant satisfaction with meetings?

2. Was the activity or activities conducted at a meeting in any way associated with participant satisfaction with the meeting?

3. Was the composition of groups, in particular the job status of a group, associated with participant satisfaction in that group?

THE STUDY

The study was conducted in a large automotive parts plant in the United States between January 1984 and May 1985. The plant, employing approximately 1700 people, makes chassis components for a variety of automobile styles. The plant is organized into two autonomous manufacturing areas, Area A and Area B, with central management and staff acting as a resource and setting major plant policies (Figure 1). Area A manufactures components of rear axles and assembles them. Area B manufactures and assembles suspension and drive train components.

Because of the decentralized nature of the plant, it was possible to form separate and decentralized ergonomic organizations in each manufacturing area of the plant. There was a total of four groups that regularly met in the ergonomics organization (Figure 2). Three of the groups were directly involved in job redesign while the fourth group served a

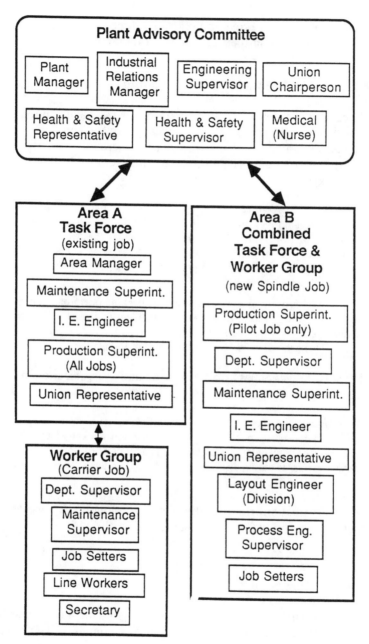

Figure 2. Plant ergonomic task force organization.

governing role, setting program policy and directions. Below is a summary of the groups and their functions within the program.

The Ergonomic Program Governing Group

The advisory committee is made up of top management and top union officials from the plant. Their function was to set and continually monitor all goals and policies of the ergonomics program.

The Area A ergonomics effort is a participative organization made up of two groups:

> *The Area A task force*—made up of middle management and area union representatives, their major responsibilities were to monitor and steer the Area A ergonomics efforts, in particular the Area A worker group, into areas of excessive ergonomic risk, serve as a clearinghouse for job redesign proposals, and provide resources for implementation of the accepted proposals.
>
> *The Area A worker group*—composed of machine operators, supervisors, and skilled trades, their role was to identify stressful jobs and determine ways to redesign the workstation to reduce or eliminate stress. This group analyzed an existing job in the plant.

The Area B ergonomics effort is a participative organization made up of one group:

> *The Area B combined task force and worker group*—combining the resources and personnel from the task force and worker group, their role was to conduct all the activities and functions of the task force and worker group as outlined for Area A. This group analyzed a new process in the plant.

The two evaluation criteria outlined above, ergonomic knowledge and participant perceptions, were measured and analyzed in the following way:

Ergonomic Knowledge

Over forty participants were trained in an ergonomic short course by a University of Michigan expert in the field of ergonomics. The training format varied between four and eight hours, was lecture-based using traditional lecture methods with extensive use of visual aids (slides, video tape, etc.), and was attended by persons who volunteered to participate in the program. They were heterogeneous in nature, representing a variety of disciplines within the plant.

Two testing methods, slides and traditional true/false questions, were used to test two types of ergonomic knowledge. The slides tested the trainees' abilities to recognize the degree of ergonomic stress on a job. Ceci and Liker[9] refer to this as nonacademic knowledge. Nonacademic knowledge is the sophisticated mental process one goes through when, for example, a carpenter measures, cuts, and assembles building material when constructing a house. Studies show that regardless of scores on IQ tests, persons are capable of conducting these activities with a great deal of accuracy.[10,11] This ability is important when one analyzes jobs and can be indirectly measured, with respect to ergonomics, by asking trainees to rate the degree of stressfulness depicted on a slide that simulates real job stresses.

A series of slides were shown before and after the training that characterized different levels of stressfulness for each joint of the upper extremity, e.g., shoulders, elbows, and wrists. Participants were asked to rate each slide on a scale of one to five, five being most stressful. The ratings were compared to those of experts in the Center for Ergonomics at The University of Michigan and given a formal score in percent correct by slide. Details of the scoring procedure appear in Joseph.[12]

Traditional true/false questions concentrate on the trainees' abilities to memorize factual information. Factual information, or what Ceci and Liker[9] refer to as academic knowledge, is often important when persons apply certain ergonomic principles requiring the use of specific facts. For example, redesigning jobs that require using and interpreting ergonomic models (e.g., the static strength model) requires a working knowledge of the model, its inputs, and the limitations of the output. This information is only known through working and knowing factual information. Approximately 20 true/false questions were administered before and after the training.

Demographic information was gathered on each person participating in the training and completing the quiz. The information included, among other things, years of industrial experience, education level, and training type. The scores for the quiz were averaged for all participants for each series of joint slides (by joint and total) and for the true/false-multiple choice questions. The data was stratified into levels by each source of information. Data analysis included comparing levels for each strata on pre-training and change between pre- and post-training quiz scores. It was hypothesized that because of the traditional lecture format of the training, persons with more formal education would be expected to perform better on the true/false questions. Likewise, persons with more industrial experience would be expected to perform better on the slide portions of the quiz. Analysis performed between level of education and years of industrial experience revealed no correlation. Therefore, collinearity between the two variables was not addressed.

Participant Perceptions

Three data sources contributed to the analysis of participant perceptions. The outcome or dependent variables of participant perceptions was based on assessments taken immediately after the meetings using a self-administered form. Eleven attributes of participant perception which were related to satisfaction of the meeting were assessed by the form. They include:

- Goals of meeting
- Goals of next meeting
- Participation of individuals
- Participation of group
- Participant knowledge of discussion topics
- Quality of decisions made at meeting
- Diagnosis of ergonomic problems
- Individuals' influence on the meeting
- Leadership at meeting
- Satisfaction with the meeting
- Satisfaction with program

The independent variables were formed primarily by using data collected during direct observation of each meeting and by using the participants' demographic information collected during the training. Meeting observations, made by the author who attended all ergonomic meetings for over a year, resulted in the creation of the variables: meeting attendance and meeting activity. As discussed in the introduction, participant satisfaction may be affected by absenteeism and it was hypothesized that higher absenteeism would result in lower participant satisfaction.

It was also hypothesized that certain meeting activities are inherently more satisfying to perform than others. However, in order to run an effective ergonomics meeting, specific activities must be performed before other activities can be initiated. Therefore, it is important that all members of the group realize the importance of all the activities. This analysis should determine what activities are and are not satisfying to participants during meetings, helping ergonomic program coordinators

TABLE I.   Percent Correct on Pre- and Post-training Quiz Scores by Question
Type (all persons who completed training and both quizzes, N = 43)

Question Type	Pre-training Scores (S.D.)	Post-training Scores (S.D.)	Percent Change
Shoulder slides	77.6 (6.5)	79.8 (7.4)	1.38
Wrist slides	66.5 (8.9)	73.4 (8.2)	6.9**
Elbow slides	68.2 (8.5)	68.5 (10.5)	0.3
All slides	70.8 (4.9)	74.1 (5.9)	3.3**
True/false	81.7 (13.4)	90.7 (13.1)	9.0**

  * significant at 0.1 level, paired t-test
 ** significant at 0.01 level, paired t-test
S.D. = Standard Deviation

to anticipate problems in meetings associated with less enjoyable activities, and make these activities more enjoyable.

Job status information, collected during the training, was correlated with participant satisfaction. It was hypothesized that certain levels of job status are inherently less satisfied with participative programs than others. Organizational literature exists supporting the fact that some industries attempting to implement participative programs have had resistance from middle management. This analysis should show if a relationship between program satisfaction and job status exists in participative ergonomics programs.

RESULT

Analysis of Ergonomic Knowledge Pre- and Post-training Comparisons

Table I shows the analysis of the average quiz scores for all participants who were trained and completed both pre- and post-training quizzes. Since only participants completing both the pre- and post-training quizzes were used in the analysis, paired t-tests were used to determine if there was a significant difference between pre- and post-training quiz scores by participants. Scores are presented separately by question type, slides to assess job stress, and true/false to assess factual information. In addition, a summary score for all the slides is included enabling a quick comparison between factual and nonfactual information.

In general, there was a tendency for all participants' scores to increase immediately after the training indicating that the training was effective in increasing the general ergonomic knowledge, factual knowledge, and knowledge used to detect job stress of the participants. Statistically significant differences between pre- and post-scores were found for the shoulder (0.1 level); wrist, all slides; and the true/false questions (0.05 level).

The pre-training quiz scores, particularly the true/false and shoulder questions, were fairly high. As no one in the sample received prior formal education in ergonomics, this suggests that either a moderate level of intuitive ergonomic knowledge already existed in the plant or that the test was too easy. Because of time constraints, a proper pre-test was not run to determine if the test was too easy. However, if this was true, then all portions of the test might have equally high pre-training scores. This pattern was not found. The participants were particularly bad at rating the wrist and elbow slides prior to the training and they did not significantly improve their ability to rate the elbow after training.

A possible explanation for this pattern is that stresses to the wrist and elbow might be less intuitive to the observer than stresses to the shoulder. Analysis of experts' agreement in detecting stress for shoulder, elbow, and wrist slides, measured by correlations, shows this to be the case. Experts were in less agreement for the elbow and wrist on comparison to the shoulder.* Therefore, spotting stresses on the elbow or wrist better distinguishes ergonomic ability (e.g., more responsive to the quality of training and participant ability to use the training) than spotting the more obvious stress on the shoulder.

The Effects of Education and Years of Industrial Experience on Ergonomic Knowledge

Analysis of pre- and post-training quiz scores indicates that a considerable amount of intuitive ergonomic knowledge already exists and that participants can learn when properly trained. However, the mean scores presented in Table I hide considerable variation in individual scores. Consequently, analysis of the individual scores may provide insight into why some trainees scored better than others.

In this context, two analyses were run: 1) analysis of pre-training quiz scores and change between pre- and post-training quiz scores by education level and 2) analysis of pre-training quiz scores and change between pre- and post-training quiz scores by industrial experience. It was hypothesized that education should be related to participant's ability to

---

*Agreement was measured by correlations between rating across pairs of experts. There was stronger agreement among the experts on the degree of stress on the shoulder (average $r = 0.87$) compared to the elbow (average $r = 0.76$) and wrist (average $r = 0.61$)

answer fact-related questions, the true/false portion of the quiz, and that industrial experience should be related to participant's ability to detect stress on the job, the slide portion of the quiz.

Table II presents correlations between education and experience with pre-training and change between pre- and post-training quiz scores. In both cases, the data supports the hypothesis on pre-training differences but not on the differential effects of training. There is a significant positive correlation between scores on the true/false questions and education for the pre-training quizzes indicating that the better educated scored higher on questions testing participants' factual knowledge. However, the slide scores did not show a similar relationship, indicating that the education level was not related to participants' having the cognitive ability to analyze jobs before training. With industrial experience there is also a significant positive correlation between wrist slide scores and all slide scores. This relationship suggests that the amount of time spent in an industrial setting influences one's ability to identify ergonomic stress correctly. As expected, there is no correlation between industrial experience and factual knowledge indicating participants did not draw on abstract factual information to analyze jobs.

There was no clear relationship between education level or years of industrial experience and change in quiz score. Generally, for the slides and true/false questions, those with high school educations and less learned as much or more than those with higher educational backgrounds, and those with few years of industrial experience learned as much as those with many years. This suggests that training, in this format, can be an effective way to transfer ergonomic knowledge, regardless of experience or educational level.

Analysis of Participant Perceptions

The Relationship Between Attendance and Participant Perceptions

It was hypothesized that in a participative program, the perceived satisfaction of the program, as measured by the meeting assessment form, would be related to attendance. Table III presents correlations between average participants' assessment of meetings and attendance at those meetings. While there were few statistically significant correlations, there was a pattern of weak positive correlations between attendance and positive perceptions, 34 positive and 13 negative. In particular, the advisory committee, the Area B combined group, and the Area A

TABLE II.   Correlation of Pre- and Post-training Quiz Score with Years of Education and Industrial Experience (N = 49)

Questions	Education (Years)		Industrial Experience (Years)	
	Pre-training	Post-training	Pre-training	Post-training
Shoulder slides	−0.145	0.121	0.176	−0.149
Wrist slides	0.156	0.180	0.385*	−0.210
Elbow slides	−0.042	−0.221	0.666	0.110
All slides	0.012	0.049	0.328*	−0.131
True/false	0.311*	0.114	0.126	0.180

* (p < .05)

TABLE III.   Correlation between Percent Meeting Attendance and Meeting Assessment Scores by Group (meeting scores based on average of all participants in meeting)

		Area A		Area B
	Advisory Committee (n = 20)[a]	Task Force (n = 13)[a]	Carrier Group (n = 14)[a]	Spindle Group (n = 14)[a]
Clarity of meeting goals (Goals 1)	0.352	0.122	0.371	0.312
Clarity of goals for next meeting (Goals 2)	0.040	0.663[b]	0.080	0.230
Individual participation (Part. 1)	0.012	−0.396	0.156	0.325
Perception of group's participation (Part. 2)	−0.024	0.229	−0.112	−0.049
Knowledge relevant to discussion (Know.)	−0.249	−0.396	0.284	0.531[b]
Importance of decision (Decis.)	0.026	0.595[b]	0.248	0.097
Diagnosis of ergonomic problem (Ergo.)	0.038	0.000	0.214	0.240
Influence over decisions (Influ.)	−0.170	−0.123	−0.199	0.204
Leadership quality (Lead.)	0.289	−0.202	0.107	0.109
Satisfaction with meeting (Sat. 1)	−0.074	0.236	0.166	0.156
Satisfaction with meeting (Sat. 2)	0.667[c]	0.026	−0.155	0.120
Mean score (Mean)	0.094	0.065	0.174	0.220

[a]Number of meetings for each group
[b]Significant correlation at 0.05 level
[c]Significant correlation at 0.01 level

worker group all had high correlations between attendance and clarity of meetings (0.352, 0.312, 0.371, respectively). The Area A task force had a significant and high correlation between attendance and clarity of next meeting. The advisory committee showed a significant correlation between satisfaction and attendance (0.667), and the Area A task force showed a significant correlation between attendance and a measure of the "importance of the decision" (0.595). Finally, a significant correlation was found for the Area B combined group between attendance and the perceived "knowledge of the topics discussed" (0.531).

It is interesting that attendance was consistently highly related to the goals of this or the next meeting. Apparently, since the program stressed the participative approach, the groups felt it was important to set clear and meaningful goals when a majority of the participants were present.

Other significant correlations noted above seemed to be related to the particular group's function within the program or to the experiences within the group. For example, the reason the "perceived quality of decisions" might be highly related only to the Area A task force's attendance might be due to their role within the program. Their main functions included guiding the Area A worker group to problem areas, deciding which alternative solutions would be implemented, and providing support for the smooth and successful implementation of a project onto the plant floor. In completing these tasks, the task force membership had to include a diverse array of specialties in the plant. Absence of any member, along with the specialty brought to the group, could seriously hamper the group's capacity to make decisions concerning any of the above functions.

Likewise, program satisfaction was related to attendance only for the advisory committee. This finding was probably related to the group's membership. Close to one-half of the group was made up of managers, whose duties usually include spending a large percentage of their day attending meetings similar to those encountered in the ergonomics program, and who know from experience, the consequences of poor attendance during the launch of a program. Therefore, attendance was used as a yardstick for measuring satisfaction and success of the program.

Finally, participants' "knowledge relevant to the discussion" was significantly correlated to attendance for only the Area B combined group. The reason for this relationship may be twofold. First, since this group assumed the responsibilities of both the task force and the worker-group, they had a wider variety of duties and functions to complete at each meeting. Unlike the groups in Area A, the Area B combined group could not request information from another group. Second, they could not seek help from other areas in the plant because, as a launch team, no one in the plant was more knowledgeable about the process than members of the group. Therefore, completion of these duties depended on participants within their group having the necessary knowledge and information to complete the task and on their regular attendance at meetings.

The Relationship Between Meeting Activities and Participant Perceptions

Five generic activities were identified during active observation of meetings. The five activities are

1. *Program Maintenance*: Development of action plans and group maintenance activities.

2. *Problem Identification*: Activities involved in identifying ergonomic stress on the job.

3. *Workplace Redesign:* Redesign activities to reduce or eliminate ergonomic stress.

4. *Implementation*: Activities involved in implementing or installing the workplace redesign solutions.

5. *Nonergonomic*: Activities that are not directly or indirectly involved in the program's content or maintenance.

After each meeting, a meeting log was transcribed summarizing the main events that occurred and estimating the percentage of time groups participated in the five activities. Table IV presents correlates between the percentage of time groups devoted to each activity and the mean meeting score (average of all measures of meeting satisfaction), by meeting. The data indicate that groups responsible for workplace changes were more satisfied when a large portion of their meeting time was spent doing implementation activities. Implementation activities tended to be more informal and dynamic and gave participants a sense of accomplishment, i.e., things getting done.

However, for the group not responsible for workplace changes, the advisory committee, the data indicate they negatively evaluated meetings that were dominated by implementation activities. Early in the program, before they clearly defined their role, the advisory committee attempted to redesign and implement workplace changes. They failed to change a single job. This resulted in a careful reevaluation of the program's goals and a reevaluation of their role in accomplishing them.

Problem identification activities were generally regarded negatively by the groups despite the fact that this was a central activity for groups

TABLE IV.   Correlation between Individual Activities and Mean Meeting Score By Group (meeting scores average of all participants in meeting)

| | Advisory Committee (n = 20)[a] | Area A | | Area B |
		Task Force (n = 13)[a]	Carrier Group (n = 14)[a]	Spindle Group (n = 14)[a]
Program maintenance	0.142	−0.285	−0.054	0.060
Problem identification	−0.066	−0.186	−0.600[b]	0.229
Workplace redesign	−0.152	0.185	−0.120	0.147
Implementation	−0.421	0.477[c]	0.676[d]	0.308
Non-ergonomic activities	0.000	−0.126	0.250	−0.596[b]

[a]Number of meetings for each group
[b]Significant correlation at 0.05 level
[c]Significant correlation at 0.1 level
[d]Significant correlation at 0.01 level

making changes to the floor. To facilitate this activity, the Area A worker group developed an ergonomic checklist. This formal system may have made meetings less dynamic and frustrating for participants. On the other hand, the Area B combined group did not use a checklist resulting in a less formal job evaluation methodology, but in more dynamic meetings.

The Relationship Between Job Status and Participant Perceptions

Figure 3 presents participants' perceptions by job status for all groups combined. Regardless of group, middle managers had significantly lower scores than other organizational levels. This observation is important because in participative programs such as this ergonomics program, the responsibility for its success often hinges on the cooperation of the middle managers. This may have to do with the role middle management plays in traditional organizations. Frequently, they are trapped between management's expectations in having successful and innovative programs in their plants and middle management's responsibilities in meeting strict production schedules.[13] Unless there are beneficial rewards for participating in the program, it may be difficult convincing middle management to risk any time commitment in activities that are important for the program's success.

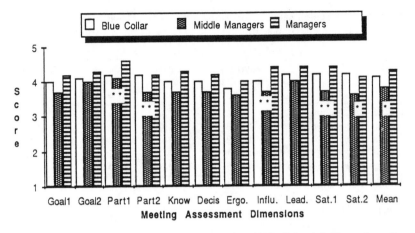

Figure 3. Meeting assessments by job status (see Table III for definitions of meeting assessment dimensions); averaged across all groups: N = 40, Blue Collar = 12, Middle Managers = 23, Managers = 5; * = significant at 0.1 level; ** = significant at 0.05 level.

CONCLUSIONS

Effective ergonomics programs must have sufficient in-house ergonomic knowledge and an organizational system to implement changes in the workplace. The results of this study indicate several important issues about training. First, lecture-based training increased participants' knowledge of ergonomics. Second, there was a considerable ergonomic knowledge base already present in the plant. Third, pre-training quiz results varied by participants' level of education and by their years of industrial experience. In particular, subjects with more years of industrial experience were more able to recognize stress on a job than persons with less industrial experience. On the other hand, persons with more education were better able to answer questions relating to factual information. Finally, there was no relationship between the level of education and the years of industrial experience and the amount learned. Apparently, the training was able to communicate equally well to all participants.

The implications of this data for training participants in future ergonomic programs are threefold. First, the existing in-house knowledge base should be used more effectively before training begins to assess the training needs. Second, lecture-based training is an effective way to train participants, but the instructor must be aware that the most important knowledge base for these new practitioners is often a combination of personal experience and the information from the training. Third, ergonomic knowledge alone cannot cause significant ergonomic changes in the plant. If it could, the existing ergonomic knowledge base should have resulted in better ergonomic designs. Consequently, there must be some concerted effort to organize persons with the knowledge for it to be utilized effectively.

The results of this data also indicate several important issues about the organization. First, participative organizations are effective in reducing the communication barriers that prevent persons with relevant knowledge and interests from working together. However, if these organizations are to remain effective, the goodwill and commitment of the participants must be taken into consideration. Second, maintaining a high level of attendance at meetings is important. Failure of members to attend meetings adversely affects the performance of the groups. Third, some activities are less enjoyable but important to the success of the program. Finally, job status may affect participant perceptions of the program. In particular, middle management were less likely to find the program satisfying.

REFERENCES

1. Westgaard, R.H. and A. Aaras: The Effect of Improved Workplace Design on the Development of Work-Related Musculo-Skeletal Illnesses. *Appl. Ergonomics*, pp. 91–97 (June 1985).
2. McKenzie, F., J. Storment, P. Van Hook and T.J. Armstrong: A Program for Control of Repetitive Trauma Disorders Associated with Hand Tool Operation in a Telecommunications Manufacturing Facility. *Am. Ind. Hyg. Assoc. J. 46*:674–678 (1985).
3. Liker, J.K., B.S. Joseph and T.J. Armstrong: From Ergonomic Theory to Practice: Organizational Factors Affecting the Utilization of Ergonomic Knowledge. *Human Factors in Organizational Design and Management*, H.W. Hendrick and O. Brown, Jr., Eds. North-Holland Publishing Company, Amsterdam (1984).
4. Hall, D.T., D.D. Bowen, R.J. Lewiciki and F.S. Hall: *Experiences in Management and Organizational Behavior*, 2nd ed. John Wiley and Sons, New York (1982).
5. Pasmore, W. and F. Friedlander: An Action Research Program for Increasing Employee Involvement in Problem Solving. *Admin. Sci. Q. 27*:343–362 (1982).
6. Hackman, J. and G. Oldham: *Work Redesign*. Addison-Wesley Publishing Co., Massachusetts (1980).

7. Maier, N.R.F.: Assets and Liabilities in Group Problem Solving: The Need for an Integrative Function. *Psychology Rev.* 4:239-249 (1967).

8. Janis, L.L.: Group Think. *Psychology Today*, pp. 6, 43-45, 46, 74-76 (1971).

9. Ceci, S.J. and J.K. Liker: Academic and Non-Academic Intelligence: An Experimental Separation. *Practical Intelligence: Origins of Competence in the Everyday World*, R.J. Sternberg and R.K. Wagner, Eds. Cambridge University Press, Cambridge, England (1986).

10. Super, C.M.: Cognitive Development: Looking Across at Growing Up. *New Directions for Child Development: Anthropological Perspectives on Child Development*, Vol. 8, pp. 59-69. C. Super and S. Harkness, Eds. (1980).

11. Fahrmeier, E: Taking Inventory: Counting as Problem-Solving. *Quarterly Newsletter of the Laboratory of Comparative Human Cognition* 6:1. S. Scribner, Guest Ed. University of California Center for Human Information Processing, San Diego (1984).

12. Joseph, B.S.: A Participative Ergonomic Control Program in a U.S. Automotive Plant: Evaluation and Implications. Ph.D. Dissertation. University of Michigan, Ann Arbor (1986).

13. Kanter, R.M.: *The Change Masters*. Simon and Schuster, New York (1983).

CHAPTER **12**

Selection of Power Tools and Mechanical Assists for Control of Occupational Hand and Wrist Injuries

ERNST VanBERGEIJK, BSME

Power Tool Section, Body & Assembly Operations, Ford Motor Company, Dearborn, Michigan

BACKGROUND

In the mass production process, many power tools are used to assemble components. Most operators in an assembly plant use power tools to complete their tasks. The occurrence of cumulative trauma disorders (CTDs) of the upper extremities is often blamed on the power tools which is one thing that most operations have in common.

Ford Motor Company (Ford) has taken various actions to reduce the potential causes of CTDs. However, before these are addressed, a brief review of the complexities of power tools would be in order.

There are a large variety of power tools available on the market, each serving a specific purpose. Ford has categorized them into five major function groups, namely:

1. Drilling
2. Threaded fastener securing (rotation)
3. Linear motion securing
4. Abrasive material displacement
5. Miscellaneous tooling

Each function group has been subdivided and a tool type designation code assigned to each type. Within each type there are a variety of sizes available (horse power/torque output) and many different suppliers.

All this information has been compiled in the *Ford Portable Power Tool Manual* as a specification and buying guide (Figure 1). A recap of the manual contents is shown in Table I. Currently, the manual contains 392 pages which is a count of the different types of tools. The number of tools reflects the various suppliers approved for each type. An average of only 2.4 suppliers have passed Ford's stringent requirements and obtained approval to sell specific tools to Ford.

The *Ford Portable Power Tool Manual* has been established for assembly and manufacturing operations only, and many types of power tools are not included in this manual. Most notable is the absence of any impact or ratchet wrenches, which are used extensively in many assembly operations other than Ford. The reason will be discussed later in this chapter.

Tools used in other industries are also available in a great variety, such as pavement breakers and chain saws. All these tools are commonly referred to as "power tools," but their variety is almost infinite.

To put Ford's power tool use into perspective statistically, Table II lists the average tool inventory in an assembly plant. There are 4,500 tools in the average plant at a replacement cost of around three million dollars. As can be seen from Table II, the vast majority of the tools used are nutrunners, and most of Ford's efforts have, therefore, been directed toward improvements in this type of tool.

CERTIFICATION PROGRAM

Ford started to take a closer look at power tools in the late 1960s, because there was trouble controlling torque within the tolerance band needed for fastener size reductions. A "Power Tool Certification Program" was initiated which requires tools meet strict performance specifications. Tool evaluation was taken out of the assembly plants and into a laboratory where the tools could be studied under controlled conditions.

The main purpose of the "Certification Program" was the development of tools with improved performance characteristics. The influence of the operators on obtaining the correct torque was found to be significant and better tools would not necessarily provide more consistent torque. Therefore, human issues had to be addressed as well.

Since the inception of the Power Tool Certification Program in 1970, many actions have been taken which enhanced ergonomics. These actions can be divided into five major areas: 1) weight, 2) torque, 3) vibration, 4) force, and 5) posture.

TABLE I.   Ford Portable Power Tool Manual Base Number Index

Section	Tool Function	Type Designation	Descriptions	Total Pages	Total Tools
I	Drilling	A	Pistol Grip Drills	11	64
		AA	Right Angle Drills	9	35
			Subtotal	20	99
II	Rotational	B	Straight Nutrunners	19	30
	Securing	C	Pistol Grip Nutrunners	61	107
	(Threaded	CA	Right Angle Nutrunners	76	175
	Fasteners)	CB	Ratchet Wrenches	0	0
		CC	Multiple Motors	38	137
		CD	Pistol Grip Impacts	0	0
		CE	Right Angle Impacts	0	0
		CF	Crimp Nut Tools	1	1
		CR	Crowfoot Tools	41	90
		CW	Tubenut Tools	14	35
			Subtotal	250	575
III	Linear	D	Hogringers & Clinchers	11	14
	Motion	E	Staplers	7	10
	Securing	H	Riveting Tools	20	49
			Subtotal	38	73
IV	Abrasive	K	Horizontal Grinders	19	43
	Material	KD	Die Grinders	9	31
	Displacement	L	Vertical Grinders	21	47
		LA	Right Angle Sanders	17	35
		M	Orbital Sanders	6	18
			Subtotal	72	174
V	Various	S	Miscellaneous Tools	12	25
			Grand Total	392	946

TABLE II.   Ford Assembly Plant Average Tool Inventory

74.8%	Nutrunners
11.4%	Drill Motors
5.8%	Abrasive Tools
3.4%	Blind Riveting Tools
1.1%	Hog Ring and Staple Tools
3.5%	Miscellaneous Other Tools

Weight

Evaluation of the physical parameters of a tool such as weight, grip size and position, balance, etc., have been part of the Tool Certification Program since its inception. Many modifications have been made and several tools rejected.

The Certification Program and competitive pressures have spawned new generations of power tools from all major tool suppliers. These suppliers have resident or consulting ergonomics experts.

To neutralize tool weight, many conventional spring or air balancers are in use in all the plants. In 1978 Ford started the development of balancing and manipulating arms for use underneath the vehicle. Over 60 of these arms have been supplied to various assembly plants, and several plants have ordered them on their own.

Three major suppliers of these types of devices are

1. D.W. Zimmerman, Inc., Madison Heights, Michigan
2. General Industrial Equipment, Pontiac, Michigan
3. New-Matic Industries, East Detroit, Michigan

The latter two suppliers use an "Erector Set" concept which makes the custom design for a specific operation relatively easy. The manipulating arms are also used for material handling tasks such as fuel tank decking, door installations, etc.

Torque

The exposure to torque reaction has two main components, namely the force of the reaction and the time of exposure to that force.

Torque Reaction Force

To limit the torque reaction force, which has to be absorbed through the operator's hand, specifications and actions are:

- Specification of reactions bars on straight tools over 28 in.-lbs and pistol grip tools over 60 in.-lbs (1971).
- Maximum force from right angle tools — 60 lbs (1974).
- Develop torque-absorbing overhead balancers (1973).
- Develop tool-mounted nut holding devices (1978).
- Develop tool support and reaction arm for pit operations (1979).

The use of torque-absorbing devices is limited by accessibility and manipulation restrictions. Acceptance and use of these devices varies greatly between plants.

Torque Reaction Time

The length of time an operator is exposed to the maximum reaction force is controlled by the operator if a "stall" tool is used, as the operator has to release the trigger. On "shut-off" (T) tools, the speed of the shut-off mechanism controls the time.
Specifications and actions are:

- Specify the use of T tools over 30 ft-lb (1973).

- Measure reaction force and impulse (lbs-sec) for right angle tools over 14 ft-lbs and list values in the Power Manual (1977) (Figure I).

- Specify the use of T tools for all sizes (1979).

Vibration

All Ford-certified power tools use a rotary air motor with gearing, which have minimal vibration. To reduce vibration exposure on other power tools, the actions to date have been:

- Eliminate the use of piercing hammers (1971).

- Eliminate specification of impact wrenches (1972).

- Eliminate specification of ratchet wrenches (1973).

- Abrasive tool evaluation at free speed and maximum horsepower. Vibration was one of the criteria for rejection (1982).

- The University of Michigan (U. of M.) has developed instrumentation to measure vibration transmitted to the operator. Evaluation of impact wrenches was completed in August 1985. The data showed that the exposure limit, based on the I.S.O. 5349 (1980) proposed hand and arm vibration exposure guidelines, was exceeded by the conventional impact wrench for total daily occupational exposure greater than 30 minutes. This scientific study showed that the decision made 13 years ago to ban the use of impact wrenches has avoided many potential causes of CTDs.

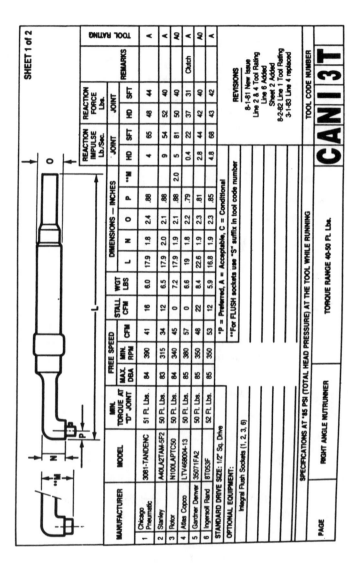

Figure 1. Sample page from the Ford Portable Power Tool Manual.

Force

The push force required to start a fastener and keep the drive bit or socket engaged during the securing cycle can cause ergonomic concerns. Most of these are created by the design of the vehicle or the fastener. Actions taken to minimize these are

- Guidelines for feasibility review were published in Operating Procedure III-A-30 (1978). Among these are limitations on cross recess fasteners as the push force required increases with torque, provide clearance for reaction bar-type tools if possible, and use multiple spindle nutrunners where possible.
- Request release of self-reacting fasteners to eliminate use of back-up wrench which often puts the operator in an awkward posture (1981).
- Increased broach depth on "TORX" recess drive specifications (1984).
- Initiated a program to reduce the specifications and use of drill point screws (1984).

Posture

Awkward postures are caused by a combination of tool selection, job allocation and vehicle design.

Tool Selection

There are hundreds of different tools listed in the Power Tool Manual. For a given torque specification, the choice of tool configuration is six different types with a choice of up to eight suppliers within each type. Selecting the optimum tool for an operation must be done on the assembly floor as the operator posture must be determined.

Job Allocation

Working height, combination of operations, movement, etc. have to be considered. Education of plant personnel to be conscious of ergonomic considerations is required.

The educational process has been addressed aggressively at Ford during the past two years. The Body & Assembly Division has a contract with The University of Michigan's Center for Ergonomics to provide research, evaluation assistance, and education. Hundreds of people from our division have attended seminars at U. of M., and many sessions have been conducted at Ford assembly plants.

The association with U. of M. has been very beneficial as the science of ergonomics has provided quantitative measurements for the elusive term of "common sense." Several of the power tool suppliers have attended their excellent seminars, which has increased their awareness and understanding of ergonomic issues.

CONCLUSION

Vehicle reliability and ergonomics go hand-in-hand. Reduction of stresses and strains on the human body will reduce the potential for incorrectly performed operations. Power tools and fasteners are a major part of the assembly process and over 50% of our workforce is affected by them.

There are, however, some misconceptions among the people not closely associated with power tools and the assembly process. These are:

- Power tools are a major cause of CTDs.
- Power tools must be redesigned to eliminate CTDs.

Both these statements are *incorrect* as far as the assembly process at Ford is concerned. Ford uses many power tools, but the time element for the operator of the actual use of the power tool is only a fraction of the overall cycle time. Each operator repeats the same task roughly 60 times per hour. Most operators secure less than three fasteners within their one minute cycle. Each fastener takes less than one second to secure. The exposure to the maximum torque reaction force is less than 20 milliseconds. In other words, the actual use of the power tool is less than 3% of the operator's cycle time while the exposure to the maximum tool reaction force is less than 0.1%. The remaining 97% of the time is used for manipulating parts and the tool.

There is no conclusive evidence that any of the tools Ford currently specifies for assembly operations are contributing to CTDs. The design of the tools could be improved in some very specific instances, but overall the tools are adequate.

It is the way the tools are being used that creates ergonomic concerns rather than the tools themselves. The proper selection of the tool type in relationship to the operation to be performed is the key, but there are always trade-offs to be considered. For example:

- Providing a manipulating device will relieve the operator of tool weight and torque reaction, but it will restrict the free movement and add mass to be moved around.

- Selecting a right angle tool over a pistol grip or in-line tool often requires two hands on the power tool.

- Adding a reaction bar to a tool to absorb the torque will eliminate the tool reaction forces but increases the weight.

Through careful selection of the power tool for each operating station and providing external assisting devices to minimize the stresses and postural problems, occupational CTDs can be minimized. It takes well trained individuals with in-depth knowledge of power tools and the assembly process to obtain optimal benefits.

Strength Test Protocol Work Hardening Study

RICHARD E. JOHNS, Jr., M.D., MSPH

A. Environmental Conditions

1. All environmental distractions must be minimized. Temperature and lighting conditions should be standardized, noise should be reduced by closing doors to the testing area, and spectators or other study participants should not be allowed in the testing area.

2. The subject should be dressed in loose, comfortable clothes suitable to perform full range of motion of the upper and lower extremities.

B. Examiner Instructions

1. The examiner should carefully explain to the participant the purpose of this research study, what the equipment is designed to test, and explain the minimal risks involved with muscle strength testing, e.g., mild muscle soreness, muscle strain, or the remote possibility of a ruptured low back disc.

2. The examiner should have the participant sign the human subject consent form, and then sign and date under the witness signature block.

3. The strength test worksheet should be initiated giving subject biographical data, date and location of test and test conditions. All test results must be entered after each position tested.

4. The examiner should provide positive, general verbal feedback to the

subject; but during the testing procedures, restrict specific performance values from the subject to avoid uncontrolled competition
between subjects.

5. The examiner should give no subjective impression of how the subject
performed, as each subject is his own control. He should be told that
he did "just fine" and that "he is not being compared to other individuals in the group."

C. Strength Testing Procedures

1. Static Strength

   a. Positions:

      1) Lift—arms flexed (red)
         Shoulder—Neutral
         Elbow—90° Flexion
         Hips—Neutral
      2) Lift—shoulder high/arms flexed (yellow)
         Shoulder—45° Forward Flex
         Elbow—90° Flexion
         Hips—Neutral
         Knee—Neutral
      3) Lift—torso stooped over (blue)
         Shoulder—Neutral
         Elbow—Neutral
         Hips—75° Flexion
         Knee—Neutral

   b. The patient should be instructed to step up on the platform and
   place his feet in the position marked with red tape. The examiner will move the handlebar height to the position marked
   with red tape.

   c. The subject will then be asked to grasp the handles and to
   perform a practice exertion in that position by gradually exerting resistance against the handles until he feels he has reached a
   maximum safe exertion for that position.

   d. After the patient has practiced this position test one time, he
   will then be requested to perform three exertions for each position as listed above, and marked for foot and handle position
   by red, yellow, and blue tape.

   e. For each exertion, the peak and three-second time-averaged exertion levels will be recorded by the computer. These values will then be recorded onto the strength test worksheet by the examiner.

    f. There should be a 30-second rest period between each exertion.

    g. After a two-minute rest period, the patient will be instructed to perform the following dynamic strength tests.

2. Dynamic Strength Testing (as above)

    a. Positions:

        1) Lift — arms flexed (red)
        2) Lift — shoulder high/arms flexed (yellow)
        3) Lift — torso stooped over (blue)

    b. The patient will be instructed to perform a practice dynamic lift of ten pounds under the direction of the examiner.

    c. He will then request that the examiner add additional weights until he feels the load to be lifted in each of the above three testing positions represents his safe lifting maximum.

    d. The examiner will record the final weight on the strength testing worksheet. There is no time-averaged value for this test, only the peak weight which the subject achieves.

    e. There should be a 30-second rest period between each dynamic exertion and between each test position.

    f. At the conclusion of the test, the examiner should thank the patient for his participation and tell him that he can find out the results of this research study by writing Cottonwood Hospital after it has been completed sometime in the late fall.

Index